A Change of Plans

A CHANGE *of* PLANS

Women's Stories
of Hemorrhagic Stroke

SHARON DALE STONE

SUMACH
PRESS

To my sister Jan.
Hard as it was for me, I know it wasn't easy for you either.
And to the memory of my parents, Adela Kobelka and George L. Stone.
They were there for me in important ways.
And to any woman who has survived a stroke
only to feel alone — I've been there.

LIBRARY AND ARCHIVES CANADA CATALOGUING IN PUBLICATION
Stone, Sharon Dale, 1955-
A change of plans : women's stories of hemorrhagic stroke /
Sharon Dale Stone.

Includes bibliographical references.
ISBN 978-1-894549-65-3

1. Intracranial aneurysms — Patients — Biography. 2. Brain —
Hemorrhage — Patients — Biography. 3. Women patients — Biography. 4. Women
with disabilities — Biography. I. Title.

RC388.5.S86 2007   362.196'8100922   C2007-901470-4

Edited by Lisa Rundle
Designed by Liz Martin

Sumach Press acknowledges the support of the Canada Council
for the Arts and the Ontario Arts Council for our publishing program.
We acknowledge the financial support of the Government of Canada through
the Book Publishing Industry Development Program (BPIDP)
for our publishing activities.

ONTARIO ARTS COUNCIL
CONSEIL DES ARTS DE L'ONTARIO

Contents

ACKNOWLEDGEMENTS 7

A CHANGE OF PLANS: AN INTRODUCTION 9
A Note on Health Care Systems

DEIRDRE FRAMPTON 27
Finding a Purpose: The Value of "Otherness"

LAUREN MAYES 45
Travels in Little-Known Worlds:
The Quest for Education

LIZ HOLTBY 65
Bloody-Minded Despite It All:
Disempowerment and Depression

ESTHER STEIN 83
Re-Imagining Oneself:
Self-image and Abuse

CHRIS MADSEN 105
An Unusual Right-Handed Person:
Disability and Identity

KATHERINE PRICE 121
Adjusting to a New Future:
Independence and Dependence

VICKY EVANS 141
The Importance of Feeling Genuine:
Career and Identity

CINDY DAVIS 158
The Best Thing that Ever Happened:
Attitude and Acceptance

IDA KING 173
Learning to Laugh at Yourself:
Living with Impairment

VIOLET CARBERRY 195
Lemons into Lemonade:
The Role of Support

JEAN BARTON 211
The Joy of Singing:
Rehabilitation

EPILOGUE 231

GLOSSARY 237

SELECTED INTERNET RESOURCES 245

Acknowledgements

I am delighted to publicly thank those who, in various ways, have been involved in the production of this book and who have helped to shape it. Most of all, I thank the women profiled here, who took the time to talk to me so openly about their experiences and who so readily responded to my post-interview questions about details as I was writing their stories. I hope that you find this book as satisfying to read as I found it satisfying to learn about your life, and I hope that you will rejoice in knowing that others will now be able to learn from your experiences. Special thanks go to Ida King who generously offered me a bed for the night when I travelled to her home to interview her, and to the parents of Deirdre Frampton who went out of their way to make it possible for me to spend time talking to Deirdre. Had they not insisted that I was welcome to stay the afternoon and night at their home, and then insisted upon driving me to a different town the next day, I would not have been able to manage fitting a visit with Deirdre into a tight schedule.

I am grateful to the Social Sciences and Humanities Research Council of Canada for granting me funds that allowed me to travel and interview women in various places in Canada, the United Kingdom and the United States. The funds also allowed me to hire research assistants who helped me with transcribing, organizing and analyzing the large amounts of data that resulted from the interviews. I thank the following women who worked in this capacity: Christine Blackburn, Karli Brotchie, Elizabeth Dubois, Katja Maki, M. Ahmeda Mansaray, Kristina Marcellus, Satnaum Mead and Sasikala Nair. Each worked on portions of the data — sometimes just a little, sometimes a lot — and each offered insights into the data that ultimately enriched my own understanding. I am grateful to all of you. Thanks also to Dr. Chris Wallace at Toronto Western Hospital, who assisted me with finding survivors and with getting ethical approval from the University of Toronto.

Thanks to Wayne Antony for his interest in this book and for putting me in touch with Beth McAuley at Sumach Press. As I have worked on writing and revising the book, Beth's excitement has been gratifying. Thanks, Beth, for all you've done in making this book possible. Lisa Rundle, my editor, has been enthusiastic and encouraging as she worked to help turn my sometimes disjointed ideas into a coherent manuscript. With an outsider's perspective, Lisa could see things that were not so obvious to me. I thank her for the careful attention she brought to this project, for affirming the value of what I wrote and for helping to make this book stronger than it would otherwise have been.

The person who played the most crucial role in making it possible for me to write this book is my partner, Sophia Gubbins. Throughout what I call my "survivors project" she has been by my side to listen to my ideas and offer her own insights. Her constant willingness to intellectually engage with me has been exciting, productive and sustaining. Equally important, she has graciously put up with being a "writer's widow" while simultaneously taking over many of my domestic duties so that I could spend time writing. Sophia, thanks for being who you are, thanks for your support and thanks for working to provide me with creature comforts so that my writing process was more pleasant than it otherwise would have been. Thanks also to my son, Mickie, for nourishing my spirit by being the delightfully loving boy that he is and for understanding that I couldn't always play with him as much as he wanted.

A Change of Plans:

AN INTRODUCTION

I begin this collection with my own experience of hemorrhagic stroke. I do not want it, though, to be the centre of attention. Rather, I want you, the reader, to understand why putting this book together has been my passion for more than a decade. To understand that you need to know something about what happened to me.

The year was 1967. Canada's centennial, San Francisco's summer of love. At the end of August, I was a month shy of my twelfth birthday, living on the outskirts of Montreal with my parents, my younger sister and younger brother: too young to appreciate the significance of the summer of love going on somewhere out there, but I remember my mother taking me and my siblings to see Canada's Centennial Train when it arrived in nearby Dorval. I remember the trips to the Expo 67 World's Fair in Montreal, as various members of the extended family came to stay with us, and I remember my excitement and anticipation over starting high school in September.

In 1967, the Protestant school system in Quebec was reorganized so that high school would begin in Grade 7. To me, high school represented maturity and no longer being a little kid. The school was far enough away that I would be taking a bus to get there, and to me that represented an exciting step away from dependent childhood. I was eager to get started on this new stage of my life, but as it turned out, my entry into high school would be delayed, and the new stage of my life that began that September was not at all what I had been expecting.

The evening of Thursday, August 31, was much like preceding evenings. Before going to bed, my younger sister and I played with cut-out dolls and paper clothes that we had made. I had come up with the designs myself and was quite proud of my creations. When it was time for sleep, we stowed our playthings away under the bed. Before long we were both asleep in the bedroom that we shared.

Around two in the morning, I woke with an incredibly painful headache. If I try really, really hard, I can catch fleeting snatches of my memory of this, but they are vague. I don't recall being frightened or thinking that there was anything unusual going on, because I was used to getting bad headaches, having been plagued with them for as long as I could remember. I think I also have a real memory of staggering to the bathroom to get some Aspirin. Although I might be mixing up the memory with some other occasion, I know that I did this because that's what my father says I told him when he asked me what happened. I have no sustained memory of anything that took place over the next few weeks. Only intermittent glimpses, and I am no longer sure whether these images are real or stories I've told myself. It was, after all, nearly forty years ago.

I don't remember returning to the bedroom that night, but that's where I was found after my sister raised the alarm. She woke to find me throwing up in bed. She woke our parents in the next room and they came running. They found me unconscious, lying in a pool of vomit. My father says he tried to sit me up and bring me around, slapping my face repeatedly. Apparently, this caused me to open my eyes and moan, but I was like a rag doll and could not sit up on my own. So he bundled me in the car and took me to the emergency department of the local hospital while my mother anxiously waited at home with my sister. My little brother slept peacefully through it all in his own room.

At the hospital, I am told, the doctor surmised that I had taken sleeping pills rather than Aspirin (this, despite my father's protests that I had no access to sleeping pills), so I had my stomach pumped. Fortunately, I was not conscious for that. Apparently, I was also fed a large quantity of strong coffee, but I remained largely unresponsive. After several hours, with no signs of improvement, the doctor decided that I had the flu. My father was told to take me home and, perhaps because he thought I just might still have drugs in my system, get me to walk around as much as possible. I was not to be allowed to go back to sleep during the daylight hours.

Two days later, to abridge what happened next, I had gotten worse instead of better and was taken by ambulance to Montreal Children's Hospital. I was seen by a team of neurologists and, after a lumbar puncture (to check for blood in my spinal fluid) and two arteriograms (the definitive test for a brain hemorrhage, which involves injecting dye to make blood vessels visible), I was diagnosed as having had a subarachnoid hemorrhage on the brainstem. This was in the days before CT scans became commonly used to find brain abnormalities. A subarachnoid hemorrhage is a type of brain hemorrhage, and a brain hemorrhage is a type of stroke.

I'm not sure when I became aware of this diagnosis, as I remained mostly comatose for several weeks afterwards. I imagine that at some point my parents must have told me what happened, but I'm sure that in my semi-conscious state, it must have been meaningless to me. The entire right side of my body had been paralyzed, but I don't recall wondering about what had happened or wondering what would happen to me. I don't recall being distressed about not being able to move my right side. I do recall that it was a tremendous effort to talk, so I said as little as possible.

I remember little about the seven weeks that I spent in the hospital, and I gradually returned to a normal state of consciousness. Mostly what I remember is that my mother spent the mornings with me, but she had to return home at lunchtime to be with my little brother when he came home from kindergarten. I remember that the nurses were always interested in collecting and measuring my urine, but this was not easy to do because half the time I wasn't aware of needing to pee, and in any case, peeing into a bedpan was easier said than done given that one side of my body was paralyzed. As often as not, I would miss the bedpan, so my mother used to sing to me (to the tune of "Twinkle, Twinkle, Little Star"), "Tinkle, tinkle in the pot, we don't want to miss a drop!" I also remember being taken to a special room in the hospital on my birthday so that I could see my siblings — in 1967 children were not allowed as hospital visitors (rather ironic considering it was a children's hospital). Once, though, my father and a nurse conspired so that he could sneak my little brother in to see me.

Towards the end of my stay in the hospital, I began therapy to relearn how to talk, walk and, generally, to use my irrevocably changed body. The therapy intensified after I returned home — daily physical and occupational therapy continued for months. I recall the physical therapy being quite painful because I was required to try to move my paralyzed right side. I hated it, and if it had been up to me, I probably wouldn't have participated. But my mother was unrelenting in her insistence that I work at my exercises. Slowly at first, and then more quickly, I regained some ability to will my arm and leg to move. I was able to walk unassisted after a few weeks. I learned to become left-handed, as no one believed I would ever be able to recover my right-sided fine motor skills (they were right, I never have). After I had been home for about a month, I was visited by Miss Walker who had been my Grade 6 teacher, and Mr. Duffel who was to be my Grade 7 homeroom teacher. They were there to assess my academic abilities. I'll never forget how awkward I felt being the centre of attention for these esteemed visitors. Once they agreed that my cognitive skills had not been damaged, arrangements were made for me to do catch-up work at home and then return to school in January, going in the afternoons only. I finished Grade 7 that way. By the beginning of Grade 8, I had recovered most of what I would ever recover, and I went to school on the same basis as everyone else. Finally I had made it to high school and, as far as I was concerned, my stroke was ancient history that was not to be talked about.

Ever since the stroke, I have not been able to use my right side very well, have poor balance, tire easily and have subtle yet troubling cognitive difficulties. At the time, my parents were assured that my intelligence had not been affected, and this is true, but in high school I began to be aware of difficulties with understanding abstract concepts. I had a terrible time trying to understand geometry; algebra, no problem

— it's so logical — but geometry, I just didn't get it! When I went to university as a young adult, I became aware that I could not follow an argument unless it was laid out very precisely — my brain simply could not fill in the missing pieces. (It's quite amazing, therefore, that I became an academic and that abstract concepts are my stock in trade, so to speak.) Other cognitive difficulties include poor short-term memory. I can't give a talk without notes, for example. No matter how well I may know what I'm talking about, without my notes I'll forget what I want to say, or I'll repeat the same point over and over. As for putting two thoughts together when I'm tired — forget it!

Nevertheless, it was almost twenty years before I stopped denying to myself that I had significant physical disabilities, or that I had been psychologically traumatized. I knew, of course, that I had impairments — I was aware of them on a daily basis — but I saw them as difficulties to be overcome, or at least hidden as much as possible. I lived in fear that someone would actually see how hard it was for me to perform an everyday task such as buttoning my clothes. If a friend boasted of putting herself through school by waitressing, I remained silent, not wanting to admit that I didn't have the dexterity to be a waitress. I learned early that people only see what they are prepared to see. If I talked about the stroke at all — and I rarely did — I made light of it: a serious illness in the distant past with no lasting consequences. I grew up in a family that didn't talk about adversity or psychological trauma of any kind, and I absorbed the attitude that there was no sense crying over spilt milk. I didn't process my stroke experience as a child, because I was led to believe that there was nothing to process.

My attitude began to change in the 1980s as I became acquainted with disability rights activists and the concept of ableism. I began reading the then nascent disability studies literature, and I learned to see my impairments in a new light, from a perspective that does not value "able" bodies over "disabled" bodies and does not regard impairment as something to be overcome but rather as a part of what it means to be human. I became involved with the DisAbled Women's Network and was outspoken about disability rights. I began to see the extent to which the physical environment is arranged to exclude disabled people, and how that arrangement works to send the message that disabled people are not valued members of society. Yet, I was mostly associating with or reading about others who were visibly disabled. My own impairments were by and large invisible to other people. My new disability consciousness allowed me to stop acting as though my impairments were something I needed to overcome, but I knew of no one else like me. It was hard not to feel isolated in my experience.

I had heard of others who had survived a brain hemorrhage, such as the actress Patricia Neal who had a hemorrhagic stroke in 1965, and I knew, theoretically, that it could happen at any age, but I had never heard of it happening to anyone else as young as I had been (later, I learned that stroke in childhood is considered rare, but no one really knows how often it happens — current estimates put the incidence rate between 1.3 to 13 per 100,000 per year).[1] It was not until the 1990s that I began to truly appreciate that I was not the only young person ever to have had a stroke. Once I realized that, I was able to begin looking at the psychological consequences of my childhood trauma, and I was able to access a righteous anger in me about the silence that had surrounded my experience. The catalyst for my new awareness about stroke in childhood and young adulthood was my discovery of a journal article by Esther Stein (a pseudonym) who ended up participating in my research for this book. She had had a hemorrhagic stroke when she was twenty-four years old, caused (as mine had been) by a ruptured arteriovenous malformation or AVM. She wrote in detail about her experiences with hospitalization, rehabilitation and recovery.

I chanced upon her essay one day while browsing the university library stacks, looking for something else. I can still see myself in that library; I remember the incredible excitement I felt as I read the title of the article, "Stroke: A Personal Perspective,"[2] and as I realized that a young woman had written it. Despite having by then a familiarity with disability theory and friendships with other disabled people, reading that article allowed me for the first time to cut through the isolation of my stroke experience. It was deeply comforting to know that what I had always thought was my unique experience was really not so exceptional.

Over the next few years, I thought a lot about the sense of shame that I had learned to develop regarding what had happened to me, along with the psychic trauma that I was not supposed to talk about but that had indelibly shaped me at a crucial time in my childhood. With my new awareness that there were others like me out there somewhere, I began to wonder how their own stroke experiences had shaped them and how they dealt with what happened. I wanted to know who they were, what happened and how they had been affected. This wondering was the birth of what I call my survivors project, which has led to the creation of this collection of survivors' stories.

I see this collection as a contribution to literature not only about women's health but also and more importantly about women's life experiences. Feminist thought has matured to the point of recognizing that women are not a homogeneous group, that our experiences are conditioned by factors such as race, class, ability, sexual orientation and so on. Categories such as these, however, barely scratch the surface of the complexity of individual women's lives. And even when we all have the same "objective" experience — in this case, surviving hemorrhagic stroke — our differences from each other can be great. The eleven stories in this book attest to that: we were affected at different stages in our life journeys; we were treated differently by health care professionals, with differing consequences for us; we have been left with different impairments and even when our impairments are similar, we have reacted to them differently; and we have all made sense of what happened in our own unique ways. This, for me, is key: each of the women profiled in this collection is an individual, with all that that implies. We share womanhood, we share survivor status and we share a determination to get on with life, but we may share little else. I see this collection, then, as a celebration of the different ways in which women come to acknowledge the role of hemorrhagic stroke in making them who they have become.

The Basics

In trying to understand what happened to the women profiled in this book, it is helpful to understand something about hemorrhagic stroke, its diagnosis and its treatment. I must caution, however, that the information I present represents my own understanding only. While I have researched these issues extensively over the past decade, reading many scholarly articles in medical journals, and am confident that I know what I'm talking about, I am not a physician; I am not an authority on these issues. I am someone with a vested interest in understanding what happened to me. Please note also that a glossary of the medical terms I use throughout the stories can be found at the back of the book along with a selection of Internet resources.

Thanks to public-awareness campaigns in recent years, most people have heard of strokes and have a vague awareness that strokes can kill or permanently disable, but this tends to be the extent of their knowledge. Few are aware that, even though older people are more susceptible than younger people, it is not uncommon for a person of any age to have a stroke. Even babies can and do have strokes. Moreover, when a young person has a stroke, it is quite likely to be hemorrhagic — approximately 20 percent of all strokes are hemorrhagic, but that rate jumps to more than 50 percent of strokes in people under the age of fifty.[3]

There are two types of stroke: ischemic (pronounced: is-skeem-ic) and hemorrhagic (hem-mor-a-jic). Ischemic stroke is what happens when arteries to the brain become blocked, usually by a blood clot. This causes severely reduced blood flow and the oxygen supply is cut off. Ischemic stroke can be caused by a variety of factors, but women who smoke and/or take the birth control pill increase their risk of developing blood clots, which can cause an ischemic stroke. Hemorrhagic stroke is what happens when there is bleeding in the brain, and this is often, though not always, caused by a ruptured aneurysm. An aneurysm is a weak spot in a blood-vessel wall and it may be congenital (present at birth) or it may be an abnormality that develops as a person ages. For aneurysms that develop after birth, there is some evidence that smoking, drinking and high blood pressure play a role, but there is at present no way to definitively point to a cause. Approximately 6 percent of the general population is thought to have a brain aneurysm, but very few aneurysms ever rupture, and there is currently no way to accurately predict which will rupture and which will not. Of aneurysms that rupture, however, the majority do so in people over the age of thirty. Women appear more likely than men to suffer from a ruptured aneurysm and hormonal factors seem to play a role, but the association remains unclear.

Another but less common cause of a hemorrhagic stroke is a ruptured arteriovenous malformation. An AVM, which is essentially a tangle of blood vessels anywhere in the body, is always congenital. As with aneurysms, there is no way to accurately predict whether an AVM will rupture, but evidence indicates that it is likely to rupture at an earlier stage of life. A study of the general population in the New York City area found a mean age of thirty-three years for detected cases of brain AVM hemorrhage.[4]

A ruptured brain aneurysm, AVM or other brain malformation such as a cavernous malformation, causes blood to spill into the brain, and this is called a subarachnoid hemorrhage. The term refers to bleeding between the middle-membrane covering of the brain and the brain itself. Specifically, it occurs within the cerebrospinal fluid-filled spaces surrounding the brain (also known as the subarachnoid space). Another type of hemorrhagic stroke is called intracerebral hemorrhage. In this type of stroke, a blood vessel in the brain bursts and spills into the surrounding brain tissue, damaging cells, and this appears to be primarily caused by high blood pressure. Intracerebral hemorrhage is the most common type of hemorrhagic stroke. Interestingly, incidence studies in the United States show that Black people are far more likely than white people to have both kinds of hemorrhage, though it is not clear why this is the case. There is a high mortality rate associated with hemorrhagic stroke, with estimates as high as 60 percent.[5]

Diagnosing a hemorrhagic stroke is not necessarily a straightforward process because symptoms can vary significantly. Typically, someone who has had one will experience an excruciating headache, will vomit, lose control of one side of the body and lose consciousness, although not all of these symptoms are always present, as the stories in this book show. In any case, when doctors suspect that someone may have had a hemorrhagic stroke, there are several diagnostic tools available. Since the 1970s, it has become common for doctors to use a CT scan — an X-ray that gives cross-sectional images — but even this tool will not always show that there has been bleeding in the brain. Other procedures, used prior to the widespread availability of the CT scan and which are still commonly used because they can so clearly show the location and the extent of a bleed, include the lumbar puncture — the insertion of a needle into the lumbar region of the spine to withdraw fluid and look for the presence of blood, and the angiogram (also known as an arteriogram) — a procedure whereby a catheter is placed in the blood vessels leading to the brain and a contrast agent or dye is injected to give detailed pictures of the blood vessels.

There are various options for treating subarachnoid hemorrhage due to a ruptured aneurysm or AVM. Sometimes, surgery can be performed to clip the aneurysm or remove the AVM, to ensure that it will not rupture again. Sometimes, it is also necessary to have a shunt inserted to drain fluid away from the brain. Increasingly, aneurysms and AVMs are also being treated with less invasive procedures. For aneurysms, a process known as endovascular embolization involves inserting coils into the aneurysm to block blood flow, while the embolization of an AVM involves injecting a glue-like substance into the blood vessels to block blood flow. An AVM may also be treated with high-intensity radiation, a process known as radiosurgery, which destroys the abnormal blood vessels. Finally, a ruptured aneurysm or AVM may be treated conservatively, which means that the survivor is placed on strict bed rest and watched carefully, but no other treatment is performed. This is the least common option chosen. There are ongoing debates among neurologists and neurosurgeons about what the best treatment is, but it is clear that one cannot unilaterally be considered superior. The best option always depends upon a multitude of factors. For some, this may mean surgery, and for others, this may mean no treatment.

Disabling Consequences

The consequences of hemorrhagic stroke depend on where in the brain the stroke is located, how much bleeding there is and how long the bleeding lasts. Sometimes, for those who undergo surgery to repair an aneurysm or AVM shortly after a hemorrhage, there are no lasting impairments. More often, even those who have surgery in a timely manner sustain residual impairments. Sometimes they are relatively minor, such as the loss of a sense of smell or taste, but even prompt and appropriate medical attention cannot always prevent impairments that significantly interfere with the ability to negotiate daily life in the way one did before the stroke.

Common consequences include cognitive impairments (especially difficulties with memory or aphasia, a type of language or speech impairment), hemiplegia (one-sided paralysis), motor impairments (especially one-sided weakness that can make it difficult or impossible to perform tasks requiring fine motor skills), difficulties with maintaining balance (so that it would be difficult or impossible to walk a straight line), impaired senses (especially vision, but touch and smell are also commonly affected) and susceptibility to overwhelming fatigue (so that it becomes difficult or impossible to function). As well, those who survive a ruptured aneurysm or AVM are often left with epilepsy. Generally, epileptic seizures are caused by scarred brain tissue that can periodically interfere with the transmission of electrical impulses of the brain.

Regardless of the type of stroke, a survivor can potentially be left with one or all of these deficits. Even though hemorrhagic stroke and ischemic stroke can have similar consequences, hemorrhagic stroke is typically more disabling than ischemic stroke because hemorrhagic stroke causes bleeding that can spread to different areas of the brain, whereas ischemic stroke is contained to one part of the brain.[6]

Gathering the Stories

Although hemorrhagic stroke affects both women and men, I chose to interview women only. In part, my decision is based on my own judgement that I would be able to identify more closely with women, and to draw on my own experiences as a girl and then a woman in order to ask questions and make sense of responses. A second reason for interviewing women only, however, is a more political one. That is, there is a growing academic literature about the experience of surviving stroke, but this literature rarely highlights the issue of gender. When women's experiences are discussed, they tend to be subsumed under those of men. For example, the issue of return to work for young stroke survivors is gaining attention, but there is no gendered analysis of how the concept of work can represent different things to women and men — women, for example, are typically responsible for housework and childcare in addition to paid employment. The question of the difference that gender makes is largely ignored. A focus on women only, therefore, is a way of positing women's experiences, rather than men's, as normative. We women are trained to recognize the ways in which our life experiences are similar to those of men. This can make it hard for us to recognize and honour the ways in which our lives are different from those of men. A focus on women only allows both women and men to appreciate what surviving stroke can look like from women's points of view.

Between the years 2000 to 2005, I travelled within Canada and to various places in the United States, England and Scotland, to interview each of the eleven women whose stories are collected here. The women were between the ages of eight and forty-nine at the time of the stroke, and they ranged from nineteen to fifty-seven at the time of the interviews. Each interview participant was at least three years post-stroke; for two women, it had been more than thirty years. I first connected with these women in a number of ways: some responded to a notice I placed on an Internet site for those who had had an aneurysm or AVM; some responded to a notice I had placed in a newsletter for young stroke survivors; one responded to a letter that her physician had sent out on my behalf; and four were survivors I had read about and subsequently set out expressly to find. I told all of the women that I was both an academic researcher and a survivor of childhood stroke, and that I wanted to write a book about their experiences. I also told them that the research had been approved by my university's research ethics board, and in the case of a woman contacted through her doctor, the hospital's research ethics board. Not everyone I contacted was able to participate; for example, the feminist filmmaker Bonnie Sherr Klein, who had had a stroke in her forties, was in the process of writing her own story when I contacted her (and her book was subsequently published).[7]

Generally, my question for each of the women was: "How have you been affected by having had a stroke?" I did not have a prepared list of questions going in to each interview. Rather, my questions arose in response to what each woman had to say during the course of the interview. There were, however, a number of issues that I tried to cover in each conversation, and if the woman did not spontaneously address an issue, I asked her about it. These issues revolved around recovery and rehabilitation; being a medical patient; being or not being recognized as disabled; self-image; relations with family, friends and co-workers; and perceptions of the significance of the stroke in terms of being a life-changing experience. There was also space for the women to talk about anything else they considered important.

The Survivor's Perspective

In the medical literature, we survivors are almost always referred to as patients. Sometimes, we are called sufferers. From my perspective, though, these terms are objectionable. We are not patients in a hospital or otherwise under constant medical supervision; not one of the women in this book would claim that "suffering" is a good term to define her experiences. It is more accurate to say that we are survivors, because we have not only survived a stroke when many have not but we have also gone on to make a life for ourselves — full lives in which we have made room for our impairment.

In telling these survivors' stories, my intention is not to give an "accurate" or "objective" rendition of what is involved in surviving a stroke. Rather, I am interested in representing each survivor's subjective perspective. Quite possibly, we survivors "misremember" things, focus on things that others consider insignificant, ignore things that others consider highly significant or otherwise do not "get it right." Nevertheless, what concerns me is each survivor's experience of it all, how she made sense of what happened and how she has (or has not) integrated remembered experiences into her life since the stroke.

A Change of Plans is a collection of stories about lives in process. I interviewed each woman at a particular point in time, so what they had to say in the interview is not necessarily what they would say to me now. Rather, the stories they told me were the versions of their lives they were comfortable sharing with me at that specific moment.[8]

Moreover, it is important to appreciate that, in the words of the feminist educator Leslie Rebecca Bloom, they continue to "grow emotionally and intellectually and continue to make important choices about their lives after the researcher has ceased to 'document' these choices and changes."[9]

I have written these stories based on what each woman was willing to tell me about her experience. They represent the sense that *I* have made of what they had to say. Each woman has seen and approved what I have written, with the exception of two. These two women have not seen what I have written about them because, unfortunately, I have been unable to maintain contact with them. I do, however, have their written consent to write their stories based on the interviews, and I think they would endorse how I have written about them.

I have also quoted most of the women quite liberally, so that their own words can be read and so that we can gain insight into how they talk about what happened. At the same time, I have done some work to "clean up" what they said. As the narrative researcher Jane Elliott explains, this means I have removed most of the "extra verbal material captured on the research tape such as ... repetition, false starts, and non-lexical utterances such as 'umms' and 'errs.'"[10] I have not, however, *completely* sanitized the quotes. I think it is equally important to show that the women were talking about their experiences in a way they had never talked about them before, and that meant that they sometimes repeated themselves, contradicted themselves or rushed to make a new point before fully explaining the previous point. I have worked to maintain a sense of this texture.

The very fact that women told their stories to *me* — an interested and sympathetic survivor — surely changed, if only subtly, how or what they thought about their experiences. For most of the women, talking to me represented the first time they had ever talked to someone else about their experiences in an in-depth way. Thus, the interview was an occasion to reflect on and articulate things that they may not have previously thought about. Similarly, what they had to say in correspondence with me, or in the interview, was influenced by their understanding of who I was and why I was interested in their stories. I, as both researcher and sister survivor, was very much part of each interview, shaping it with my questions, my responses to their questions and my responses to what they had to say.

I've arranged the stories in order of the interviewee's age when the stroke occurred. To some extent, how each of us dealt with what happened or came to terms with the consequences was a factor of how old we were at the time. Yet it would not be accurate to say that our experiences were determined by our ages. Nor would it be accurate to say that the younger we were, the more traumatic the experience was. The degree to which we were traumatized, I would say, is related to what we were dreaming about for the future, and what it meant to us to have to change those plans.

We all have a story about the actual stroke event, getting medical attention (some of us got prompt attention, others had to wait quite a while before being taken as seriously ill) and getting rehabilitative therapy (again, some of us got quite a bit of therapy, others didn't get the therapy they needed). Where we differ most is in what we did after health care professionals were done with us. Some of us quickly took our newly acquired impairments in stride and made new plans, most of us railed for years against the perceived injustice of being denied the opportunity to realize cherished dreams. Each of us has a unique story to tell about how we were affected.

I have written each story to highlight one particular theme, and at the same time I have strived to give enough detail of each woman's life so it is understood within her specific circumstances. Themes explored include feeling "other," education, anger and depression, self-image, abuse, disability and identity, independence and dependence, the role of support, attitude and acceptance, living with impairment and issues to do with rehabilitation. But within these, many additional themes emerged as the women talked about their experiences, including faith, motherhood, romantic relationships, financial resources, work and career, loss, isolation and invisible impairments.

I suspect that some readers might find it strange that I use the term "impairment" rather than the term "disabilities." Indeed, none of the women I interviewed used the term "impairment"; rather, they all used the more common term "disability" when discussing their abilities or lack of ability. Nevertheless, I use impairments in an effort to highlight that impairment is a bodily state that is not necessarily negative. People with impairments become disabled in situations or in the larger society when things are not arranged to accommodate impairment. This is a disability studies perspective that clearly identifies the most significant challenges arising outside the individual.[11]

*

Each woman's story appears under a pseudonym and anyone else mentioned has also been given a pseudonym. To further protect the identities of these women, I have also declined to mention where exactly they live, beyond the country of residence. Where relevant, I note whether she lives in a rural or urban environment. I wanted participants to feel totally free to discuss their experiences.

I hope that this collection will be of interest to any professional who works with stroke survivors or anyone who cares about a stroke survivor, and that it will be useful in helping to understand some of the issues that survivors deal with on a regular basis. More importantly, though, my hope is that survivors themselves will find this book both interesting and empowering. Many of us who were young when we experienced a stroke find that there is no place in Western society to talk about how stroke has changed us, and this lack of interest is disempowering. Social mores mean it can be difficult to talk about illness experiences generally — many people tend to become distinctly uncomfortable discussing illness or disability in other than abstract terms. It is especially not easy to talk about going through an experience that most people know nothing about. One risks being dismissed as unintelligible. Thus, I hope that survivors, especially those who feel isolated in their experience, will find something in these pages with which to identify and thereby feel a little less strange.

NOTES

1 John Kylan Lynch, "Cerebrovascular Disorders in Children," *Current Neurology and Neuroscience Reports* 4 (2004), 129–138.

2 Since Esther wishes to remain anonymous, details about this publication are withheld.

3 Bradley S. Jacobs, Bernadette Boden-Albala, I-Feng Lin and Ralph L. Sacco, "Stroke in the Young in the Northern Manhattan Stroke Study," *Stroke* 33 (December 2002), 2789–2793; Heather Bevan, Khema Sharma and Walter Bradley, "Stroke in Young Adults," *Stroke* 21 (March 1990), 382–386.

4 Christian Stapf et al., "The New York Islands AVM Study: Design, Study Progress, and Initial Results," *Stroke* 34 (May 2003), 29–33.

5 Azita G. Hamedani et al., "A Quality-of-Life Instrument for Young Hemorrhagic Stroke Patients," *Stroke* 32 (March 2001), 687–695.

6 Ibid.

7 Bonnie Sherr Klein's *Slow Dance: Story of Stroke, Love and Disability* was published by Knopf Canada. It is now out of print, but paperback copies can be obtained by contacting the author directly at bklein@dccnet.com. In 2006, she released her documentary *SHAMELESS: The ART of Disability* through the National Film Board of Canada.

8 See James A. Holstein and Jaber F. Gubrium, *The Active Interview* (Thousand Oaks, CA: Sage, 1995).

9 Leslie Rebecca Bloom, *Under the Sign of Hope: Feminist Methodology and Narrative Interpretation* (Albany, NY: State University of New York Press, 1998), 94.

10 Jane Elliott, *Using Narrative in Social Research: Qualitative and Quantitative Approaches* (Thousand Oaks, CA: Sage, 2005), 52.

11 Terminology is always a political issue, and it should be noted that, even though this perspective is dominant in the field of disability studies, there is not unanimous agreement on how to understand either impairment or disability. It is far beyond the scope of this book to review the debates, but the interested reader might want to compare Simi Linton's arguments in *Claiming Disability: Knowledge and Identity* (New York: New York University Press, 1998), and Shelley Tremain's philosophical treatment of the issue in her article "On the Government of Disability," *Social Theory and Practice* 27, no. 4 (October 2001), 617–636. As well, Shelley Tremain has recently put together a thought-provoking collection on the application of the thought of Michel Foucault to the study of disability: *Foucault and the Government of Disability* (Ann Arbor, MI: University of Michigan Press, 2005).

A Note on Health Care Systems

The stories in this book offer a somewhat international perspective on how medical care is organized and experienced. The women were variously treated in Canada, the United States and the United Kingdom. In Canada, citizens are entitled to free basic health care, which includes visits to a physician, hospitalization, physician-ordered tests and rehabilitative services, such as physiotherapy if ordered by a physician. Mobility aids such as wheelchairs, canes or crutches are not covered; neither are prescription drugs. Those who are employed sometimes have health care insurance as an employment benefit, to cover all or a portion of the costs not paid for by the government. Regardless, there are no restrictions in Canada in terms of which physician an individual may see or which hospital she/he may go to. The Canadians in this book (aside from myself) are Lauren Mayes, Vicky Evans and Violet Carberry.

In the United States, health care is mostly privatized, which means that there are few public hospitals and people are expected to buy health care insurance. Those who are employed sometimes have health care insurance as an employment benefit, to pay for all or a portion of costs associated with illness. Employed Americans are likely to be covered by a system of "managed care" whereby individuals insured by a health maintenance organization (HMO) are entitled to the services of participating physicians and hospitals. Low-income Americans may be entitled to Medicaid, which will cover the cost of basic services at public hospitals. In the following stories, Ida King received medical services at a public hospital, paid for by Medicaid. The other American women in this book — Deirdre Frampton, Esther Stein, Chris Madsen and Katherine Price — had private health care insurance to cover most of the costs associated with their recovery from stroke.

In the United Kingdom, the health care system comprises elements similar to those found in Canada and elements similar to those found in the United States, with the unique element of having physicians and nurses employed directly by the government-run National Health Service (NHS). The system is complex, but to make sense of the treatment received by the women in this book, it is helpful to know that the comprehensive health care services provided free of charge by the NHS are rationed, and there are frequently long waiting lists. This affected the services received by the British women in this book: Deirdre Frampton (who emigrated to England), Liz Holtby, Cindy Davis and Jean Barton. Underfunding also means that many hospital patients do not receive as much attention as they might otherwise. In the following stories, this was a particular issue for Jean Barton. There is also a growing private health care system in the UK, with physicians who do not participate in the NHS, hospitals that are run on a for-profit basis and services provided by non-NHS professionals.

Deirdre Frampton

FINDING A PURPOSE:
THE VALUE OF "OTHERNESS"

Deirdre Frampton had a hemorrhagic stroke of unknown cause in 1991, when she was eight years old. Deirdre, who is of Anglo-Saxon heritage, lives in England where the family emigrated from California when she was nine; she was nineteen at the time of our interview. We arranged to meet in late 2002, when she would be home with her parents during her break from classes at college. Since her home was quite a distance from town, her parents graciously invited me to spend the night. Deirdre seemed quite happy to meet me, given that I, like her, had had a stroke in childhood. Her parents were pleased as well and had many questions for me about my own experiences. Deirdre didn't show the same eagerness to pepper me with questions, but I suspect that she may have felt less comfortable doing so because of our age difference — I was, after all, more or less the same age as her parents. Nevertheless, Deirdre and I were able to talk at length about her experiences, mostly in the presence of her mother. We sat together in the living room, sometimes briefly joined by Deirdre's father, who was otherwise busy preparing our supper.

Deirdre's youth means that she remains close to many childhood experiences that those who are older tend to forget. Her story is a reminder of what it can be like to be an adolescent and then a young adult. Deirdre talks about going through these formative years with significant impairments. Her story raises many issues, such as the significance of educational experiences, the power of religious faith and what happens when rehabilitation is not ideal. Above all, though, Deirdre's experience illustrates what it is like to feel "other" — not fitting in with peers, being treated as different from everyone else and feeling alone in one's experience. In many ways, Deirdre's experiences diverged from my own, but her angst over being treated as different during those crucial years of adolescence, when most of us desperately want to fit in, certainly resonated with my own.

*

At eight years old, Deirdre was a friendly little girl, full of life, always happy to do what she could to help out others. She excelled academically, and she would help her schoolmates with their homework. She was in the Gifted and Talented Education Program at her California school, designed for pupils with exceptional academic abilities. One summer day, though, she fell off her tricycle and hit her head. Although it was painful at the time, she doesn't recall feeling lasting pain from the fall. Within six or seven hours, however, she had "a massive, massive headache." She collapsed, began to vomit and to drift in and out of consciousness. Her mother carried her to the sofa, and her father, who had some police training, checked her vital signs and physical abilities. He asked her to squeeze his hand, which she could do with her left hand, but not her right. Her entire right side had gone limp. Then he checked her eyes with a flashlight, only to find that the left eye responded to the light but the right did not. Her concerned parents lost no time getting her into the car and driving her to the hospital.

Upon arrival at the hospital she was given a CT scan. On the basis of the test results, and her symptoms of right-sided hemiplegia and aphasia, she was tentatively diagnosed as having had a stroke and admitted to hospital. The doctors wanted her to have an arteriogram but they had enormous difficulty finding a vein into which they could insert the needle. After Deirdre was poked fourteen times by four different nurses, her father had had enough and would not let the nurses continue to traumatize his daughter. No other procedures were attempted.

Deirdre, for her part, mostly remembers feeling scared — she had lost the use of her right side and had great trouble speaking and writing. She wondered what was going on and why she had lost her abilities.

After four days in hospital, during which time Deirdre steadily improved, she was discharged. At this point, she was still waiting for a definite diagnosis. Upon discharge, she still did not have use of her right side, she walked with a pronounced limp and could not speak clearly. Doctors, it seemed to Deirdre's parents, were uninterested in doing anything for her. They were told in so many words not to worry, that she would recover because she was a child who was still growing. The Framptons insisted, nevertheless, that Deirdre be seen by rehabilitation experts.

Deirdre was given a referral to a large rehabilitation assessment centre, where she was seen by a physical therapist and an occupational therapist. The centre would not take her as a patient, however, because it focused on those who were barely functional. Since Deirdre was at least able to walk and talk, even though she did so poorly, she was sent home and her parents were given a long list of things to do with her to help her improve the functioning of her right side. For example, Deirdre's mother remembers that Deirdre was supposed to practice picking up clothes pegs every day and placing them on the edge of a can. Deirdre, however, refused to try. It was simply too difficult and too painful. When her parents tried to cajole her into doing exercises, she would dig in her heels and cry. About this, Deirdre said: "I have a very strong will, and when I've made up my mind about something, I will *not* do that thing, you know."

Deirdre's stroke was confirmed two weeks after discharge

from hospital when she had an MRI. Her parents explained the diagnosis to Deirdre, but she didn't really understand. All she knew was that it felt "very weird to go from one day being just an ordinary person who walks down the street to the next day being in a wheelchair." She spent the rest of the summer gradually recovering her ability to speak, and her walking improved somewhat. She tells the following anecdote about an incident that took place after she had been home for a while: "There was a girl down the street and she came around one day and she looked at me and said, 'Oh she's much better now, isn't she?' And then I smiled at her, and she went, 'Oh!' Because I could only smile with one side of my face."

She started Grade 3 in September. Before long, however, the school vice-principal called her parents to say that the teacher could not cope with Deirdre in the classroom. Deirdre, it seems, had gone from being a gifted student to being illiterate: she was aphasic, and she had no attention span. She would not, for example, sit and listen to a story but would run off and start playing with things in the room. This previously outgoing, friendly child now did not mix with the other children and would spend a lot of time crying.

At first, the school addressed Deirdre's problems by calling in an educational psychologist to deal with what they thought was depression. She would see the psychologist once a week and was encouraged to talk about her feelings. This did not help Deirdre fit in better at school, though, and she recalls being upset with the very idea of needing to go to counselling. From her perspective, it was unnecessary. Then the school authorities had her assessed in preparation for going to a special school for learning-disabled children. As a result, Deirdre was able to get some speech therapy and cognitive rehabilitation sponsored by the school district. She also transferred to the school where her mother, who was a teacher, worked; there she could get learning support and speech therapy. Deirdre remembers how much she loved her speech therapist, a warm and caring woman. She was always eager to see her for a session, during which time she would practise using nouns and adjectives, with which she had difficulty (a typical symptom of expressive aphasia). The therapist also gave Deirdre's parents tips on how to play games with her so that she could improve her ability to express herself with clarity.

Although Deirdre spent most of the school day in a regular classroom, a daily routine at school became going to the learning support centre, where she would work on academics with one-on-one support. She was required to do math, reading and writing, and many tasks were turned into games. Because tasks were geared to accommodate Deirdre's special needs, she was able to achieve on her own terms. Being able to do things helped considerably with Deirdre's self-esteem, and she loved going to see her support worker. "I used to think that was one of the best parts of the day," she said. The experience left such a strong impression on her that years later she said, "I still remember the smell of the room."

At the same time, Deirdre didn't understand why she could no longer do things that she used to be able to do effortlessly. She was easily frustrated when she could not do what she wanted. Although she liked going to the learning support centre, and she liked being with her speech therapist, she was not happy about needing this special support. Coupled with her physical impairments, her self-confidence plummeted.

She finished Grade 3, and then the family moved to England, where her father is from. Deirdre's parents were hopeful that she would get better medical treatment in England, with that country's National Health Service (NHS), than she had received from the American Health Maintenance Organization (HMO). Upon arrival in England, Deirdre was registered and put on a waiting list for physical and occupational therapy. She waited about two years for services from the NHS, after which point her parents realized that unless they paid for services themselves, she was not going to get what she needed.

At age eleven, Deirdre started going for physiotherapy, which her parents paid for. She was by then old enough to appreciate the benefits of trying to use her right side, even if it wasn't easy. She especially liked playing with a big ball that she was supposed to roll on to help strengthen her leg which was turning outward. She rarely did the exercise as she was supposed to, however, and she soon stopped doing other exercises as well. She went for weekly sessions for about six weeks, and then she stopped going. In part, she stopped going because it was difficult for her parents to manage paying for the therapy, but there also seemed little reason to continue to pay for it, as Deirdre was not committed to working at her exercises. She saw no point. Not only was it difficult for her, but she had also become used to not being able to do things. She thought she would manage just fine without therapy. In hindsight, she said that she didn't realize that by not working to use her right side, things would get worse. Indeed, over the years her foot became deformed because of walking on it improperly, and her hand became cramped to the point that she could not open her fingers.

Perhaps Deirdre was also put off going for physiotherapy because of how the physiotherapist treated her:

> I can remember her taking me outside and this was the first time that I really noticed that I had a limp, because she said, "Right, walk in a straight line down there," and she had my parents standing with her and she said, "You see, look, you know, look at her, look at her walk." I really felt as if I was being ostracized then 'cause she says, "OK look, look at her walk there, oh look, look, can you see?" And then she did sort of an imitation of me. And I thought, that's not very nice. But it wasn't exactly how I walk, it was a bit more than how I walk, and she said that, but I thought, still, that's not very nice to do in front of an eleven-year-old girl, walk how she walks. You know, with a limp.

Up until that point, Deirdre had not thought about how she appeared to others. The incident caused her to start becoming conscious of how she walked, stood or generally used her body. She did not think there was anything wrong with how she did things, but she did not want to be singled out as someone who was different. So, she made a conscious effort to be aware of how she used her body and tried to do things so that no one would notice her differences.

School, meanwhile, was not a pleasant experience for Deirdre. Although she got some help with academics, she did not get as much as she had had in California. She found it very difficult to cope with her schoolwork. On top of that, she was bullied and teased by some of her schoolmates not only because she spoke with an American accent but also because she limped and had a "funny arm" (she used to hold her arm up with her elbow bent, which is very common with paralysis or hemiplegia as muscles have a natural tendency to contract).

After a boy she was playing with told her that she "ran funny," she decided to ask her father to tell her whenever she was holding her arm up, so that she could become more aware of what she was doing. It was difficult to always be aware of her right arm, because it had become so natural for her to hold it up. She did learn, though, to grab her right hand with her left in order to hold it down and make her look more "normal." Eventually, clasping her hands together while sitting became second nature for her.

By the time she started high school, Deirdre had gained the confidence to talk back to those who persisted in tormenting her. Once, a group of boys walked behind her, limping and holding their arms up in imitation of her. She got so fed up, she said, "I just turned around and said, 'I had a stroke, *okay*!!! How would *you* like that to happen to you?" The boys thought that was funny, though, and this gave them cause to start calling her an old lady because strokes were what happened to old people.

Deirdre found situations such as this to be very demoralizing. She put up a good front, in the sense that she exuded a friendly, even bubbly personality, but in private she often found it difficult to cope with everything. The worst thing, from her perspective, was that she needed special help to do her schoolwork, and even with such help, she still could not do well. She would compare herself with the students she saw at school who were achieving high marks, and she would think about how if she had not had a stroke, she too would be a high achiever. She knew she wasn't stupid. She was, in fact, quite intelligent. Her cognitive impairments, though, prevented her from expressing what she knew inside her head. Her cognitive impairments meant that she was labelled as a special-needs student, and she absolutely hated being a special-needs student.

When she was sixteen and preparing for her General Certificate of Secondary Education (GCSE) exams, she became fearful that she would not pass. One of her friends impressed upon her how important it was to pass the exams, going so far as to say that their entire futures depended on how they did on the exams. Deirdre came home from school that day in tears, convinced that her life was ruined because she couldn't hope to pass them. She did pass the exams though, and she is proud of her achievement. She was also delighted that she would finally be able to put her hellish school experiences behind her.

The next step was to figure out what she was going to do with her life. In the back of her mind, she had long thought that she would like to be a teacher. Her difficulty with academic work, however, meant that she would have to let go of that dream. She also thought that she might like to be an actress, but she wasn't sure how to go about pursuing that, considering that she was disabled. She started to think that she was a loser who would never be able to do anything.

Despondent, she prayed to God for guidance. Prayer was not a new thing in Deirdre's life. Actually, she said that she had become a Christian when she was four years old, and her faith had remained constant throughout her life. So, when she found herself feeling that everything was just such a struggle, and she wasn't sure how she would find the resources to continue struggling, she spent a lot of time praying. Eventually, she felt that God responded to her, telling her that He loved her and had a plan for her life.

Even though her faith told her that God loved her, and that He would not let her down, Deirdre remembers being amazed to learn that God had chosen her for some special purpose in life. It was a turning point. She sought guidance from her father and her minister, both of whom suggested that she should investigate Bible College, where she could study the Bible and theology, and train for a career in practical ministry. Deirdre considered this and decided that she would really like to do that.

Deirdre attended the Bible College's Open Day where she learned that graduates found work in professional and caring professions, or with Christian churches and organizations. She found it all quite exciting and felt this was where she was meant to be. She was able to enroll in a Foundation Year course to gain the equivalent of two A levels (a requirement for entry into a degree program). After completing the course, she would be able to go on to study at the college for a university degree.

The Foundation course required Deirdre to spend two days a week learning in the classroom and another four days a week in a placement where she worked with street youth. She approached her placement with trepidation. Now eighteen years old, Deirdre was only a few years older than the youths with whom she was required to work. Contemplating the task brought up bad memories of experiencing bullying from boys in high school.

In her first term working in the placement, she watched her supervisor who, she thought, handled the boys extremely well. She felt scared that she would never be able to handle the boys with the same skill. She thought that these boys would have bullied her if it were not for the fact that she was a few years older than them. Being a youth herself, she felt vulnerable. Yet she learned a lot from her supervisor. Difficult as it was, she learned to show her strengths to the youth and to offer herself as a model for others to follow. In retrospect, she said "*that* was a major step for me to be able to work with those youth and to be able — for me to show them why I'm like I am."

She realized that her own life experiences meant that she had something to teach the young people — she had faced the challenges of the stroke and of being an immigrant, and had dealt with her cognitive and physical impairments. When she stood back and thought about what had happened to her, she wondered how it was possible to juxtapose those experiences with being happy. She *was* happy, though, and she wanted the youth she worked with to realize that even though bad things might happen in life, it is still possible to be happy. More and more, Deirdre was able to take comfort in knowing that God had a plan for her, that she could rely on God to be there for her and that the negative things that had happened to her were an important part of her life story, which God would build on. She became convinced that it was her calling to work with children and youth.

None of this is to say that Deirdre is *always* happy. Just as when younger, she continues to hide from others the extent to which she can become frustrated with her inabilities. She is, by her own account, a proud young woman, and said that her pride often gets in the way of admitting that there are things that are difficult, if not impossible, for her to do. More than once she has tried to do something rather than admit that she can't, only to fall flat on her face. It has always been important to her sense of self to pretend to others that she is just like anyone else, so that when she is faced with the fact that she is not just like anyone else, she feels discouraged. She thinks that this will probably be an ongoing theme in her life: she will go along happily, but from time to time will be confronted with her impairments and the frustration of being limited by them.

Deirdre recognizes herself as disabled. To her, it means that she is not able to do what she wants to do. For example, she once went rock climbing, but it was extremely difficult and she wasn't able to climb as high as she wanted to get. Or, she recognizes herself as disabled because she can't do her schoolwork without a considerable amount of help, and even then she can't always manage to pass her assignments. This latter circumstance makes her particularly unhappy. She keeps thinking about how she had been deemed academically gifted prior to her stroke. She finds herself comparing her present cognitive abilities with those of her schoolmates and against what she was able to do when she was very young. She is afraid of being seen as stupid, when she knows that she is not. For Deirdre, being disabled means that she is prevented from doing what she thinks she ought to be able to do.

Sometimes, Deirdre finds it difficult to have others expect her to be able to do things because they can't see her impairments. She feels inadequate at such times and dislikes having to explain that she can't always meet expectations because of her stroke. There are times, she said, when she wishes her fingers were cut off so that people would be able to see that she doesn't have the use of her hand. She also finds it quite tiresome to have to continually explain her impairments to others.

> I find it very tiring when someone asks me, "Oh, why are you limping?" And they just think that I've had a, you know, accident. Or I've hurt myself running or whatever. I say, "Oh, that," and I think, Oh, I've got to tell that story all *again* and oh my goodness! And I tell them, and they say, "Oh, I'm so *sorry.*" And it's like, don't be sorry, I just told you, you know, and it's just very tiring, having to tell the story over and over and over again. And now I've just adapted to saying, "Oh, I just limp when I'm tired." But the fact is that I always have a slight limp.

At the same time, Deirdre hates having others recognize her as disabled. She wants to be seen as "normal," not as having special needs or needing special treatment. Her friends mostly treat her as she wants to be treated, but once, a close friend at school did something that epitomized for Deirdre the patronizing attitude that she abhors. It was at college, and students were expected to carry their food trays from the tables to the kitchen. Deirdre's friend, however, told her not to carry the tray because she might drop it. Deirdre felt demeaned by this comment, along with the assumption that her stroke made her incapable of carrying a tray. She responded angrily and pointed out that there was a lot that she could do, that just because she had had a stroke did not mean that she required special treatment.

Similarly, when she got a job at a clothing store, she was annoyed to be asked whether she was capable of running a till, and whether she could manage putting clothes on hangers. For Deirdre, having others question her abilities is akin to being treated as inferior. She feels objectified. Social interaction would be much easier for Deirdre if others would acknowledge that there are many ways to perform tasks, and she is a complete human being who is capable of figuring out how to get things done. Working at the clothing store, for instance, was difficult in that many of her duties required manual dexterity, but she managed by doing things her own way. Tasks that most people would use two hands for could be done with only one hand, and she coped.

To some extent, Deirdre recognizes that her desire to be seen as an independent and capable young woman is a function of her age. At nineteen years old, she is just beginning to experience herself as an adult. She is eager to leave childhood behind. So, when someone treats her as though she is not capable, she feels demeaned. She resents being treated as though she were still a child. During her first year at Bible College, for example, she lived with a host family that included a woman who had had a brain hemorrhage herself a few years previously. Others thought this was a wonderful place for Deirdre to live, thinking that the older woman would be able to understand Deirdre's challenges in a way that someone else might not. Deirdre, however, did not find that she had a great deal in common with her. Rather, she felt patronized.

> I mean, she'd even sometimes cut up all my food. It was like, I'm not a *BABY!* I don't need it all cut up. And even though it may be help — you know, it *was* help that she cut up the food for me, it all comes under pride again. And she was a lovely, lovely lady, but the fact that she cut up my meat for me was like saying to me I'm still a child. And it was like, I'm *not* still a child, I'm a *grown*-up, you know! I'm just moving out of the house, and I'm just going off to college and things like that, so I'm in my, you know, independent and dependent stage and mature/immature, and I don't know really know where I stand and things like that. So I think it has a lot to do with that as well.

At nineteen, Deirdre had completed her Foundation Year course and was enrolled in the first year of a BA program. She was able to cope with the academic work in part because it was assessed on a pass/fail basis rather than on the basis of exams, in part because she had a special needs tutor who would help her with writing essays, and in part because she could get extra time to write her assignments. She was also eligible for disabled student support. Based on an assessment, she was offered a package that included money for books and photocopying, a mini-disc recorder for recording lectures so that she didn't have to take notes, computer programs to help her with analytical tasks and a digital camera so that she could take pictures of things she needed to remember while on her field placement.

Deirdre is happy with the usefulness of all of these aids, and she appreciates the special arrangements such as being given extra time to write assignments, but at the same time, she is acutely aware of how receiving help places her under the authority of the helpers. She fears that they will want to become involved in everything that she does, including her private life. This she especially doesn't want.

Again and again as Deirdre told her story, she returned to the thought of what she could do before her stroke, how advanced she probably would be had it not happened and how much she disliked being seen as less capable than everyone else. While she did not say so explicitly, it was almost as though she was saying that she felt cheated by her stroke because she was prevented from realizing her full potential. This is not to say that Deirdre typically dwelled on her perceived losses. Actually, she spent little time thinking about them. But when confronted with situations in which her impairments were highlighted, she had a hard time not thinking about what might have been. Sometimes, she felt quite isolated and misunderstood, as she explains here:

> Sometimes, I mean, even when we got our last paper back and I got thirty-eight on it, you know, I *even* got isolated then, or I felt isolated anyway, because I was talking to a second-year and she said, "Oh, well, all the, you know, all the second-years have been through it too, you know, all the second-years have been through failing papers and things like that and just take comfort in that." And I was like [said with an angry tone]: "No, you haven't, you haven't been in my situation, you haven't had a stroke, you haven't, you know, gone from being quite intel-ligent to not intelligent at all and, you know, you haven't been through everything that I've been through and so how can you

say that?" It was almost — so it was quite nasty of her to say that, but I know that she was trying to comfort me, and tell me that, you know, "It's OK 'cause, you know, you'll pass this paper" and things like that, and then I thought deep into it, because I thought, well no you haven't.

To some extent Deirdre has always felt that others can't understand what life has been like for her. She was quite pleased, therefore, when she found someone her own age who had also had a stroke. She said:

There's a girl on the Net who's twenty. My age. I'm nineteen now, but she's had a stroke, she had a stroke about two years ago. So we go on MSN chat. And we chat about our stroke and things like that and what difficulties we have and — so that's nice, I mean, previously I didn't have anyone who'd had a stroke, or, you know, I didn't know of anyone or anything like that. I only found out about her about three months ago, four months ago.

Deirdre's cognitive impairments certainly cause her more distress than her physical impairments. Regarding the latter, she has learned to adapt how she does things to accommodate her impairments. As well, and excitingly, she began taking Botox injections when she was seventeen to allow her right hand to relax so that she could retrain her muscles and, she hopes, get to the point where it will no longer become cramped and unusable. Botox, short for Botulinim Toxin A (and now associated with anti-aging "beauty" treatments), began to be used in the mid-1990s to help stroke survivors who have disabling muscle spasms. An injection will cause the muscles to relax, but because the effects only last for three or four months, repeated injections over a period of years are required. It is very expensive, however, which may be why it is not a common treatment.

Deirdre first heard of Botox and its benefits for stroke survivors when she applied for her driver's learning permit. She was required to get a medical assessment before getting her permit. This led her to see a specialist at a stroke rehabilitation unit who lamented the fact that children were rarely referred to him, because he was able to help them. He said that he could have done something for Deirdre had she only been referred earlier. In particular, he could have recommended Botox injections when she was younger. She could have been getting appropriate physiotherapy along with the injections, and she likely would have been able to recover the use of her hand.

In any case, Deirdre got her first Botox injection for her arm and hand when she was seventeen (paid for through the UK's National Health Service). After a few days, her hand began to loosen up so that she could flex and unflex her fingers. She says that from the beginning it has been an almost miraculous treatment. Previously, she hadn't dared to think that she would ever be able to use her hand again; she was so overjoyed that she was in tears. A year later, she also had an injection in her right leg which helped to relax her toes so that they don't cramp up in her shoes, and now walking and standing for long periods is a lot easier.

Along with the injections, she sees a therapist who teaches her how to exercise her arm and hand to retrain them. Theoretically, after three or fours years she will no longer need Botox injections because by then, she will have retrained her muscles and naturally be able to use her hand. She doesn't do her exercises as often as she needs to, though. Much as she would like to permanently retrain her hand, her impairments are familiar to her. Deirdre is not interested in making it a priority that overtakes her life. Retraining her hand would require a considerable amount of time and energy each day devoted to exercises. Deirdre is not prepared to reorganize her life to focus on her impairments, which is more or less what it would take for her to make substantial progress. Indeed, Deirdre has spent much of her life so far trying to ignore the fact that she has had a stroke. She doesn't like to talk about it; she would rather focus on what is positive in her life, or on the exciting directions that her life might take in the future.

Deirdre has travelled a long and difficult road from childhood to young adulthood. She knows that there will continue to be bumps along the way, but she has also come to a place where she is able to see that being different is not necessarily a bad thing. Certainly, she feels that her own stroke experiences give her special insight when it comes to working with troubled children and youth; had she not had the stroke she doubts that she would have pursued this line of work. In a reflective moment, she summed up her view on the significance of her stroke:

> I think it makes me unique. And different. And in previous years, I hated that. But now I quite like it. I quite like the fact that people ask me, "So where are you from?" You know, 'cause "your accent's not quite English, it's not quite American." I do get very tired of, you know, having to explain why I limp and having to explain why I sometimes can't let go of things [because of her cramped hand] and stuff but, I also think that's part of my personality, I think that ... if I didn't have my stroke, I wouldn't be who I am now.

*

It might be tempting to look at Deirdre's story and think that it is only because of her Christian beliefs and practices that she has come to recognize the ways in which her stroke experiences have enriched her life. No doubt, her faith has been important to her in helping her come to terms with what happened. Yet there is more than one road to self-acceptance and Deirdre may well have arrived there even in the absence of her faith. As other stories in this book will show, learning to see the positives that stroke can bring to a life does not necessarily require religious beliefs.

Woven throughout Deirdre's story is the theme of not wanting to be treated as different, and she felt alone in her experience. This had far-reaching consequences in many areas of her life, but it strikes me that, had she been treated with more sensitivity by medical and rehabilitation personnel, she might not have rebelled so completely against everyone's efforts to "help" her correct her perceived deficiencies. Almost everywhere she went as a child, she was greeted by people who were likely to in some way point out that she was not acceptable the way she was — there was the neighbour who was aghast to find that Deirdre's smile was lopsided, her Grade 3 teacher who sent Deirdre for counselling, the physiotherapist who parodied how she walked, the boys in high school who bullied her, the friend at college who was afraid she would drop her food tray and the landlady while she was at college who wanted to cut her food for her. I find it significant that Deirdre spoke fondly of the warm and caring manner in which her childhood speech therapist treated her, and it was with speech therapy that she made the most progress. Had others shown the same sensitivity to her feelings, perhaps Deirdre would have been motivated to work at regaining more of her former physical abilities. As it was, she mostly felt treated as a problem to be fixed. With her strong will, she reacted by refusing the terms of the debate.

That Deirdre's rehabilitation was less than ideal, however, ought not to be regarded as a tragedy that causes her to lead an impoverished life. This is what an ableist perspective would suggest, but from a different perspective it can be recognized that Deirdre has spent over half of her life learning how to live with her impairments. She is used to them. From the perspective of disability as lived experience, Deirdre's impairments are part of who she is, and that is something to celebrate.

Finally, it must be kept in mind that Deirdre's life continues to evolve. After I interviewed her in 2002, she finished her college degree. She has been happily married since 2004. She and her husband are looking forward to having children in another few years. Meanwhile, Deirdre has been training to run a marathon. She hopes to be able to organize her busy schedule to actually do it in the near future.

Lauren Mayes

Travels in Little-Known Worlds: The Quest for Education

I first met Lauren Mayes, a woman of English, Irish and Scots descent, in 1996 in cyberspace several years before I got to meet her in the flesh. She had been excited to read a short narrative I'd written about my AVM rupture that was posted online because she had had a brain aneurysm rupture when she was seventeen years old, in 1970, and she wanted to connect with me. I was equally excited to connect with her — especially because she was, like me, Canadian — and I responded immediately. We developed an e-mail correspondence that continues to this day, although we no longer correspond as frequently as we did in those early days, when both of us were all but glued to our computers, anxiously hoping for a quick response to our latest missives. We very quickly established that we had a great deal in common. In the summer of 2000, I travelled to southern Ontario to finally meet Lauren, then forty-seven, in person. In the intervening years, I had met other hemorrhagic stroke survivors, both in person and via e-mail. Still, it was exciting for me to finally be able to sit down with Lauren face-to-face to hear her story.

Lauren's story reflects many of the common themes that thread throughout women's experiences — feeling "other," inadequate rehabilitation, self-image issues and faith among them. But again and again as Lauren spoke about her experience, she returned to the significance of education and the anguish she felt over having her education interrupted. Much of her life since her stroke has centred around the desire to finish her education — something that she was never expected by doctors to be able to accomplish. She has travelled an enormous distance to get where she is now, in midlife.

*

Lauren grew up in a rural village not far from Ottawa, Ontario. She was the only girl in a family with three boys — she had an older brother and two younger brothers. In the middle of June 1970, she was seventeen and looking forward to going off to Toronto — the "big city" — for the summer, as soon as she finished her Grade 12 school year. In Canada, these were the years when there was ample government funding for youth projects, and Lauren was to work for an organization to learn how to do community development. She would be living communally with other youth from around the country. She was excited about being away from home and starting her first-ever summer job. She was planning to return to her parents' home by September, to complete Grade 13 and then go off to university. She had her life all planned out: after university she would travel in Europe for six weeks, return home, get a job, get married, have children and enjoy her life. Her biggest worry was how to convince her father that she should go to university (in 1970, the idea that girls had as much right to higher education as boys had not yet become popular). Her plans were not to be fulfilled, however, because on the very last day of Grade 12, an aneurysm ruptured inside her brain.

When the aneurysm burst, Lauren felt as if she'd been "hit with a baseball bat on the inside of my head." Her first inclination was to pass out but she struggled against that. She was on the second floor of her school, in the hallway, and she kept repeating to herself that nobody dies in the upstairs hall of the school. She made herself go downstairs; a classmate helped her to the nurse's office. The cold compress the nurse put on her head intensified the pain, and Lauren started to vomit. Her mother came to pick her up. As there wasn't a doctor available Lauren's mother took her home and called the doctor's office. When the doctor's nurse answered the phone, she said that Lauren probably had flu and not to bother the doctor. Two or three days passed; Lauren seemed to be getting worse. Mrs. Mayes was becoming increasingly worried and took Lauren to the emergency room at the nearest hospital. There, the doctor said she was probably just nervous and upset about something. Even though Lauren had been suffering continuously from a headache, he prescribed Valium and sent her home again.

In certain respects, it is amazing to consider the emergency room doctor's disastrous assumption that Lauren had simply worked herself into a state over something inconsequential. Today, there are probably few doctors who would feel entitled to be so dismissive, and there may be even fewer women who would accept it. But this was 1970, and the consumer health care movement had yet to appear. It was not Lauren the doctor was communicating with — she was barely conscious — it was her mother, and her mother had grown up in an era during which one does not question the judgement of doctors. Also, it is relevant that this took place at a rural hospital, where doctors probably saw few cases of hemorrhagic stroke, and so it would not have been something they automatically thought to consider, especially in a young person. That the doctor prescribed Valium — a tranquilizer that had only been on the market since 1963 but that by 1969 had become the top-selling pharmaceutical in the United States — makes sense in light of his flippant diagnosis. Moreover, a woman in that era (and arguably, even now) was marketed to physicians as the prototypical good candidate for Valium: someone who needed to be calmed down.

Lauren remained at home for another few days feeling more and more uncomfortable, not able to tolerate light or noise. By the sixth or seventh day, her headache began to subside, but she began to lose the use of her left side. A week after her aneurysm had ruptured, Lauren's worried parents took her back to the hospital and insisted that she be taken seriously. This doctor agreed that there was indeed something significant going on and called a neurologist in nearby Ottawa who agreed to see Lauren right away, so Lauren's parents packed her into the car for the late night trip to the city. Lauren recalls:

> I'm lying in the backseat with my mother. My father's driving with the radio on and I kept lifting up my arm, and letting go of it and saying, "Oh, good, it's still not moving." Because I was terrified that by the time we got to the hospital I'd be better and then everybody would be really ticked off at me because now it's midnight and we're driving to the city, and all. And so, every time I would do that, my father would drive a little faster and turn up the radio a little louder [Lauren laughs]. And my mother would just, you know, sigh.

In this little anecdote, we can catch a glimpse of what must have been Lauren's larger experience of feeling that it was not her place to cause trouble for others. Growing up with three brothers, she likely learned early that girls were less important than boys, and so by the time she was seventeen, it would have been second nature for her to worry that she would be found perfectly healthy and the cause of great inconvenience for her parents. As everyone later learned, though, there was indeed good cause for alarm.

Once at the city hospital, Lauren had a lumbar puncture. The test showed that there had been bleeding in the brain, and Lauren was admitted to intensive care. But she recalls feeling a great sense of relief that she would be looked after now. She woke up the next morning and was surprised by something in her bed — she lifted up the covers with her right hand and only then did she realize what she'd felt was her own left arm. She had no feeling or movement on her left side and she could no longer focus her eyes to read or follow movement. She had an EEG and an angiogram, but because of the trauma to her brain, these tests were inconclusive. The doctors decided to treat her as though she had a blood clot and put her on blood thinner medication. Giving her blood thinners was, actually, not a good thing to do; they can make things worse in the case of a hemorrhage. Fortunately, doctors also made the wise decision that she should not be allowed to get out of bed. About this, Lauren says:

> When I was first in the hospital — it was summertime — it was very hot. And I remember one of the student nurses used to be able to take me out on a walk in my wheelchair and stuff. And after a little while, a few days, they decided that wasn't good. That I should be on bedrest, and then on strict bedrest. And so they knew that there was something serious, they just didn't really know what.

Lauren's father visited every day after work. As she wasn't eating well, he would bring her a differently flavoured milk shake each time and coax her to drink it. Also, because her arms were swollen and sore from the intravenous and blood testing, and because it was so hot (this is before hospitals were air-conditioned as a matter of course) he brought bags of ice so that she could have ice packs. Her mother would come every evening after supper and many afternoons. Other relatives all came regularly. On weekends her parents brought her younger brothers, then aged seven and twelve, and sometimes the family collie — Lassie — and walk her on the hospital lawn so Lauren could watch and see her. She was later surprised when someone told her how much her mother had aged that summer — every day when she visited she was cheerful, supportive and always wore a bright colour, and Lauren had no awareness of the stress her mom was under.

Meanwhile, Lauren was fretting over her plans to go away for the summer to work. In her words:

> I couldn't understand that this was going to take a long time. I couldn't understand that I wasn't just going to get better again for a while. So my father had said I should contact the place where I was going to work. I said, "Well, no, I can't do that. Because I'll be okay." I couldn't imagine that in three weeks I wouldn't be fine.

A year later, when Lauren read the letter she had finally permitted her father to write on her behalf, she realized the depth of his despair. Her father had written that Lauren was in hospital and that they didn't know if she would walk again.

Three or four weeks later the doctors performed another angiogram that allowed them to see that she had had an aneurysm rupture and where it had happened. They began preparing to surgically repair the aneurysm. Lauren, meanwhile, was still in constant pain from a headache. So she was quite excited to finally have a definitive treatment plan which, to her, meant that the doctors would fix whatever was wrong and she would get better. She did not understand the significance of the diagnosis or the treatment.

It was another four weeks before the doctors felt Lauren was strong enough to have reparative surgery. While she waited for the operation, Lauren had the distinct impression that the adults who came to visit knew more about what was going on than they would tell her, that they were afraid for her. The day before the surgery, her uncle, to whom she was very close, jokingly assured her that there would be flowers for her no matter what, either at the hospital or at Hulse's (the funeral home her family used). When she repeated this to her mother she was appalled, although Lauren thought it was funny and in an odd way comforting. She wasn't frightened but really wished that she'd be given more information. She wondered if there was a possibility that she was going to die, but nobody would say so. She recalls wishing that someone would tell her what exactly was likely to happen, or at least what the possibilities were. If she was likely to die there were things she wanted to arrange. Her neurosurgeon told her that after Friday she'd be safe, although he didn't know exactly what would happen — either her condition would be improved, it would stay the same or things would get worse.

On the day of the surgery, she recalls being fascinated by what was going on in the operating room:

> I was in number twelve operating room, and it was all these — like, the biggest one. And, my name was up. It's like having your name up in lights. And I thought, "I'm a star! And the surgeon is the big supporting actor. That it's Mayes & Bagnell!" You take your simple pleasures, I suppose. I was just really, sort

of you know, impressed by this.

The last thing Lauren remembers was the surgeon walking in and the anesthetist telling him that she was just about ready to go. Many hours later, Lauren awoke to find the neurosurgeon sitting by her bed, and she was afraid that he had not done the operation because she had not gone to sleep. But he assured her that it was all over, that he had clamped her berry aneurysm (a common type of aneurysm, so-called because it's shaped like a berry) so that it would not leak any more, and everything had gone well. Then Lauren wanted full details about what he had done, and her doctor complied. After that, she does not recall feeling either elated or disappointed. She accepted that she was still sick, and therefore she saw it as her job to get better. The first days following surgery were difficult — she was in intensive care and in pain, though for some reason she was not allowed to have pain killers. Then, when the doctors were confident that the surgery had gone well and she was recovering, she was moved to the neurosurgery ward.

As soon as she was transferred to the ward, but before she could even get out of bed, she started sessions with a physiotherapist to help her regain use of her paralyzed left side. At first, the physiotherapist would help her to move her arms and legs while she stayed in bed. Then, Lauren remembers that the first time she was allowed to stand up, she felt surprisingly stiff and sore. At that point, she remembers thinking, "I know what it is like to be eighty, but I don't know what it was like to be eighteen." She found that thought depressing. Throughout her post-surgery hospital stay, in fact, she felt that she had to really struggle against being treated as if she were an old woman. She said:

> I remember feeling at one point that I was kind of a nuisance in the hospital because I really wanted to be able to walk. And I felt that I had to really struggle against being treated as if I was sixty. Or seventy. Which was much more where I felt the nursing staff eventually had me slated. Like I had a seventy-year-old's problems. So: "Just be a seventy-year-old, and be happy that you've got a wheelchair, and a nice walker, or something."
> I really persevered, and I really didn't want — I wanted more

than that. And they really often felt as if I was being a nuisance, and having these high aspirations.

Indeed, at one point doctors recommended that her parents find a nursing home for her, as they did not think she would ever recover enough to live independently. In addition to her left-sided hemiplegia, it also became clear that she had been left with cognitive impairments that severely compromised her ability to follow what was said to her and made it difficult for her to remember things. She had trouble understanding ordinary concepts or how to connect ideas together. She said, for example, "I could read words but I couldn't connect them. So if I read a sentence it would be like reading a shopping list or something."

Neither Lauren nor her parents, however, were willing to give up. Lauren pushed herself to get back as much physical ability as possible and, finally, after two months she was able to walk, albeit unsteadily, and feed herself, although she still couldn't cut her food. She was able to go home at the beginning of October; she'd been in hospital for nearly four months.

Much as she had looked forward to going home, Lauren recalls that it was at the same time very scary for her. The hospital had been a protected environment, but she felt that outside the hospital, she would be seen as a freak. She had almost no use of her left arm, she was unable to walk well, the left side of her face drooped, she was painfully thin, she had little hair on one side of her head (her hair had been shaved for surgery), and she had started to have seizures (a common after-effect of brain surgery, due to scar tissue that interferes with normal brain functioning).

When Lauren returned home, she could not relate to the person she had been before the stroke. In part, her disconnection from her old self was due to the cognitive damage she had sustained. When she saw her old bedroom at home, she looked around with curiosity, trying to discover who she had been. Everything seemed strange to her:

I remember thinking, "Oh, you must like blue, because you have a lot of blue. And you must like to read, because you have a lot of books on the bookshelf." Just opening my drawers and sort of discovering what sort of person I was. I didn't even feel like I'd been there before. You know, it was more like a déjà vu feeling, as opposed to something that I knew well.

She had also been away for a long time, and she came back profoundly changed. When she left, she had been an able-bodied high school student, excited about her future. When she returned home, she was a severely impaired young woman who did not seem to have anything exciting to look forward to. At least, no one thought she would ever be able to do much of anything. As for Lauren herself, she saw her family treating her as though she were the same person, trying to get her interested in her old life, but Lauren knew, somewhere deep inside herself, that she would never be the same again. She knew that whatever concerns she had had four months earlier had become irrelevant and that she had a monumental task ahead of her to rebuild her life.

Years later, she recognized that she would have benefited from professional intervention at this point, but no one ever offered her any kind of counselling. No one, in fact, ever seemed to be concerned about how she had been affected emotionally. The focus was on her physical abilities.

In this respect, Lauren's treatment was typical. The lack of attention paid to the emotional well-being of stroke survivors, whether young or old, is appalling. It would be nice to think that the overwhelming focus on physical abilities to the neglect of psychological issues is an artifact of the era, and that things are different today. Lauren herself suggested that had she had her stroke more recently, she would have had better and more comprehensive rehabilitation. But it remains the case that rehabilitation is almost exclusively focused on function. What *has* changed is that more is now known about how the brain works, and so professionals are often aware of the need to check for signs of cognitive damage. Today, a survivor with cognitive damage, such as Lauren sustained, is likely to get some help with finding ways to compensate for difficulties with understanding and expressing ideas, ability to organize things, memory and speech. But survivors remain unlikely to get counselling to help them deal with what happened on an emotional level. There still seems to be little recognition that, whatever the physical consequences, survivors have suffered an emotional trauma and need to heal emotionally, not just physically.

The next few years were miserable for Lauren. She was physically weak, continually exhausted, cognitively damaged and, even though she was on anti-seizure medication, she still had seizures that she experienced as horrible. They were "grand mal" seizures, whereby her body would convulse and sometimes she even needed to be hospitalized. To a large extent, she felt that the seizures defined her during that period, and though doctors tried a variety of medications, it would be almost ten years before she stopped having them. Looking back, she said of the seizures: "It was as if the slate was wiped clean and I had to build up all the parts again. I'd go along and then it was like turning the lights out. Gone. Too much stimulation of any sort did me in — going to a mall was impossible, that sort of thing."

She continued going for physiotherapy for nine months, at first daily and then three times a week. She asked to go back to school but the school wouldn't let her return that year. So, she tried taking a correspondence course, but realized that she would never finish the course because she couldn't read. She was particularly affronted by this, as she had been a good student before the stroke and loved to read. She also applied to go to university and was accepted, but when she realized that she had been accepted on the basis of who she *had* been, and that she really would not be able to cope with the coursework, she declined the offer.

Instead of going back to school, Lauren decided to move to Toronto to work. This was a big move for her, as she had never been away from her parents for an extended period, but she felt the need to strike out on her own and see what she could do. It was while in Toronto that her seizures became more frequent — for a while, even several times a day. Realizing that she could not live her life while never knowing when a seizure might incapacitate her, she began seeing doctors, but no one seemed able to help her get the seizures under control. At one point she even considered a temporal lobotomy to remove the scarred portion of the brain, but when she realized that this would entail having her hair shaved, she balked and did not go through with it. It was fear rather than vanity that stopped her from having the surgery. She was so frightened by the thought of anything coming at her head that she did not get her hair cut for nearly seven years after her reparative surgery.

She did find work in Toronto, although she could only ever get low-paying jobs that were not very satisfying for her. Also, she was often unable to work because of her continual seizures. Socially, she became part of a group of people that she calls misfits. They, like her, seemed to be drifting aimlessly and did not seem to fit in with mainstream society. At the time, she felt such a misfit herself that she did not feel comfortable with anyone else. She felt accepted by her new friends. Secretly, though, she felt as though she was just passing through, and she hoped that no one thought that she would never be able to better her position in life. She said:

> I really didn't know how I was going to get from where I was to where I wanted to go. I used to visit friends at universities. And I would just be so envious of the life that they had. I had no idea, because I knew that I couldn't keep up. I knew that I couldn't really, I knew that I couldn't understand. And yet, that was always the life I had expected to have. I had expected to go to university, get a job and things like that. And I just didn't know how that was ever going to come about.

Lauren felt a sense of shame:

> For a long time, I was awfully aware that I couldn't walk well. And that there's things I couldn't do well, and of course I thought everybody noticed that. But they didn't. Also I was quite ashamed of myself because I felt like I — I was a high school dropout pretty well. I mean, I had grade twelve, but that was it. And I found for me that was really important, I wanted more education.

Meanwhile, she worked as hard as she could to improve her physical abilities, her memory and her ability to read. She never gave up on her ambition to get a university education. In 1976, six years after her stroke, Lauren felt ready to try going to university. She moved to a new town in southwestern Ontario and was accepted at yet another university, but she still could not cope with the work and was forced to drop out. The next year she enrolled in college instead but soon found that this too was premature. She wasn't able to complete the year. She moved back to Toronto and got a job working in a restaurant.

In 1978, Lauren converted to the Bahá'í faith and became involved in the Bahá'í community. Shortly afterwards she moved to Ottawa in order to go to college; she had been accepted into the two-year Child Care Worker Program. This time she was able to complete the program. She felt better prepared and her reading abilities had improved. Yet, it was still a cognitive and physical struggle. She recalls, for example, that from the bus stop she had to walk across a large field to get to school, but she still had difficulty with walking, and "it was really a big undertaking every time I had to cross the field." Her program was demanding — by the end of the program fewer than half of the students who had started it were still enrolled. Lauren worked hard and while she felt like she was part of the class, it was clear to her she wasn't like the rest. But she hadn't realized that others thought so too. Before graduation one or two instructors met with each student and processed their experience with them. When it was Lauren's turn, one of the instructors asked her if she was familiar with the TV comedy *Mork and Mindy* that was popular at the time. The premise of the show was that Mork was an alien who had come to Earth to study earthlings. The instructor said that in class, Lauren was like Mork, studying the others who were like Mindy. Lauren could easily identify with this characterization, as she often felt like an alien on account of her stroke, and she often felt that she didn't really understand social conventions that everyone else seemed to take for granted.

After she graduated, she got a job in an emergency home for the Children's Aid Society. The demanding job left her feeling exhausted yet satisfied. While working for Children's Aid she made a pilgrimage to the Bahá'í World Center in Haifa, Israel. One of the things that interested her about Bahá'í was the idea of being a pioneer. Bahá'í "pioneers" go to remote areas of the world to teach their faith and to found Bahá'í communities. The prospect of pioneering in faraway places greatly appealed to Lauren.

In addition to her long-standing interest in travel, Lauren certainly felt like a pioneer herself. She likened her post-stroke experiences to having been on a long journey that no one else had taken. So, she applied to be a Bahá'í pioneer but was denied because of her epilepsy. Lauren began an "intense prayer campaign" whereby she pledged that she would pioneer if only she could be cured from being epileptic. Incredibly, she stopped having seizures. By the time she was ready to travel, she had stopped taking any anti-seizure medication (against her doctor's advice) and has never had another seizure. She was then twenty-eight.

This cessation of her seizures represented a real turning point in Lauren's life. While it's not unusual for post-stroke seizures to eventually disappear, it's not clear why this happens, and Lauren is not sure how to explain why her seizures disappeared, saying there could be different explanations and contributing factors.

Lauren didn't elaborate on what may have been contributing to her seizures, but it doesn't seem far-fetched to speculate that they stopped because she had begun to find purpose in her life. Her left-sided weakness had improved so that it was no longer as disabling as in the first few years after her stroke and had become little more than a minor inconvenience. Cognitively, the improvements were equally dramatic. Her sheer determination to improve her cognitive skills meant that she had made remarkable gains. She could read and write without difficulty, she could express herself verbally and understand conversations, and connecting thoughts was not the trial it had been in earlier years. For the first time since she was seventeen, she was able to think about more than just getting through the day, and she was able to imagine a bright future for herself. It seems more than just coincidence that her seizures disappeared as she spent more time focusing on her spirituality, and this speaks to the powerful interconnections between spiritual, emotional and physical well-being.

In 1981, Lauren spent several months in Mexico. Her experiences abroad gave her confidence that she could change her life for the better. When she returned home from that experience she made plans to settle outside of Canada as a Bahá'í pioneer. In 1982 she went to Belize in Central America. Shortly after getting there, she got a job working with a high school teaching English language and composition. After three years she got a job working for CUSO, the Canadian University Service Overseas, also in Belize, and spent the next three years working on a drug-education project. Living and working in Belize, for six years, far from all the people who knew what she had been through, she was able to create a new persona as an independent and capable woman. She found that those she met in Belize were quite willing to take her just as she was — an earnest young woman who wanted to contribute to the well-being of others.

In Belize, she realized that she had regained almost all of her pre-stroke abilities, both cognitively and physically, and she once again began to dream of getting a university degree. She decided to start slowly, by taking correspondence courses from Queen's University in Kingston, Ontario. Then, in 1988, when her contract in Belize was about to run out, she decided to return to Canada rather than renew it. In retrospect, she said, being in Central America for those six years "was a good transition between being sick and being well. And so when I came back to Canada, I felt as if I'd left my sickness behind, my inability, behind."

After such a long absence, however, Lauren was no longer sure how to be a Canadian. The idea of getting a job as soon as she returned was quite frightening. She was not sure how she would manage the culture shock. She felt that coming back to Canada would be more difficult than leaving it had been:

> I decided I would come back and go to school and use that as
> an opportunity to figure out what it was like to be a Canadian.
> And do that and see. So that's what I did and at the end of it
> I had a degree, which also, really, really was a big accomplish-
> ment for me. I was really thrilled by that.

So, at age thirty-nine, Lauren achieved a degree in sociology from Queen's University. It was a dream come true. She said:

> When I graduated from there, my mother was particularly — just totally moved. Because, in the beginning after I'd had a — everybody thought that I would need my parents' help, that I would need their care. For always. That I would never be financially independent or really able to function independently.

She wondered whether she would have gone to university if she had not first lived a different way of life in Central America. She had matured while she had been away, and she had begun to come to terms with her past.

Just how far she had come emotionally is evident from what she said about getting pictures taken for her university graduation. When she was given the photo proofs so that she could choose the one she liked best, she said:

> And, on a couple of them, you could see it, I could see quite — like this part of my forehead where the incision had been and all. And, you know, I could have chosen one of the ones which covered it. But instead I thought, "No. That's me. That's fine. That's part of who I am." And sometimes I felt, well if I could live my life again and selectively, you know, erase certain events, what would I erase? And I realized, that wasn't one of them. That there were other things ... that I guess were choices I had made and I wish in retrospect that I'd made different choices. But having the aneurysm, it's different — it speaks to a different part of me. I mean, it was really like my challenge, it was really my condition.

Years earlier, Lauren had decided that she was quite interested in working in the area of child welfare. Neither her college diploma, however, nor her newly minted BA was enough to get her the kind of job she desired. Thus, once she completed her BA, she decided that she needed a degree in social work, which she earned from Lakehead University in Thunder Bay. She found a job in southern Ontario and began her career in children's services. She changed employers in an attempt to get where she wanted, and began to feel ready to settle down in one place. She had learned to drive when she went to Lakehead and now she bought herself a house in the small town of Caledonia. Then she realized that she would be further ahead if she had a Master in Social Work (MSW) degree. She enrolled at a nearby university as a part-time student, so that she would be able to keep her job working in children's mental health.

In 1997, when Lauren was forty-five years old, she graduated with her MSW. She became restless again, and started thinking about moving to find a job closer to where she grew up. The job she had no longer excited her. She was ready to move on. But fate intervened, and she developed a friendship with a male neighbour. By the end of 1998, the friendship had blossomed into a full-fledged romance. In February, 1999 they got married.

Lauren's marriage brought tremendous changes to her life. By her own account, they were all wonderful, but this is not to say that in her earlier years she had pined for marriage — she had always been ambitious and independent. She knew that she didn't want to get married until she was mentally and physically strong and able to be independent. At some point she simply relaxed about it — she felt sure that she would marry but it would be at the right time for her. Also, she had not wanted to get married when she was younger because she had been fearful of what the stress of pregnancy might do to her and she was unsure about her ability to raise children given her impairments. Caring for herself was hard enough for at least a decade following her stroke, she didn't see how she could have possibly taken care of children as well.

Getting married in her mid-forties meant that no one expected her to begin having children of her own. In any case, her husband had three children from a previous marriage, including a daughter who lived with him at the time. Lauren became a stepmother and has developed a good relationship with her stepdaughter who has since had a daughter of her own. Lauren is close to her granddaughter and sees this as a great gift.

Lauren continues to find it challenging to perform many physical and cognitive tasks, but for the most part, no one else notices. She says: "It's probably not noticeable to anyone unless they know me well and usually only when I am very tired. So, I try not to get really tired. Then, my walking can get quite poor and I start to feel quite confused."

She tells the following story, which in many ways encapsulates the subtle ways in which physical impairment continues to affect her:

> I bought a new car a couple of years ago, and I really wanted a red sporty looking car. And I decided I wanted a red Saturn sports car but they didn't have any in red, in Sports Coupe 1, which is what I wanted, that were automatic. They only had the standard. I figured, "Oh, well. Millions of people all over the world drive standards, so how hard can it be?" So, I tried, and I tried, and I tried. And I could never co-ordinate all of the things that you needed to do. So I took it back. And so there's things like that that I encountered. You know, my husband every once in a while says, "Oh, well, maybe we'll move to Italy." And I say, "Well, you know, the big problem is, I couldn't drive."

Lauren continues to find busy environments overwhelming, such as shopping centres with their myriad lights, colours and sounds, so tries to avoid those situations. She also lives with ongoing difficulties with taking in a lot of information at once:

> Sometimes if people are giving me a lot of instructions, I just, I know that I — I can't possibly follow them. Like I need to write it down and figure it out. I think I've gotten pretty good at — people don't necessarily know that I don't have a clue of what they're talking about. And I sort of figure I'll figure it out as I need to, or I'll get a little bit of information or something, or I'll go and ask somebody else and — now I know how to phrase the question so I don't get too much information. Like the job that I have now. I'm pretty good at being able to just sort of decide, "Okay, well, don't worry about it, you know. Just do this little bit." And I have written down what I have to do next, and stuff like that. And eventually — I think I'll get it sorted out. But, it's just overwhelming to me sometimes. I know that I'm relatively bright but it's just, it's like another language sometimes. And I just really have to be nice to myself

about it. But I know that I don't have the big picture.

From the vantage point of her position as a married woman with a new family, three university degrees and a successful career, Lauren is able to reflect on the journey she has taken from the time she was seventeen and her life was so precipitously changed, saying: "It seems that I spent a lot of time trying to shape my life as if nothing had gone wrong and now am able to look back at it from a different perspective."

It was only while studying for her social work degree that she began to investigate literature about trauma and to conceptualize what had happened to her in those terms. Looking back, she asks:

> What have I accomplished in my life? Well, I went on that journey, and I came back. And, you know that kind of experience and what it demands of the person and all, it's probably akin to getting a degree. In terms of the challenge that it presents, you know, I was very aware that I had to really reconstruct an awful lot of things. I had to learn to walk and just do all those sorts of things. So, I kind of knew that I had a lot of inner strength. I've felt sometimes that — I mean it's easier to talk about when it's all over with than when you're in the middle of it.

*

Education has been an important preoccupation for Lauren throughout much of her life. Again and again in the years after her stroke, she attempted to go back to school only to find that her cognitive skills were so poor that she had to drop out again. She was determined, though, to get back on the road that she had been on before her stroke.

Education was of such monumental importance to Lauren that it wasn't until she had almost completed it that she was able to begin coming to terms with her stroke. Education, of course, is not necessarily of such importance to all survivors, but Lauren's pre-stroke plans centred around higher education, and educational attainment remained important for her post-stroke identity. For anyone who, like Lauren, finds that their cherished dreams are suddenly thrown into question as a result of stroke, it can be a daunting task to maintain a healthy sense of self.

When Lauren completed her BA at the age of thirty-nine, twenty-two years after her stroke, doors opened for her, including doors to even higher education and to well-paying jobs with financial stability. We might even say the door to her loving marriage was opened too, as she was no longer consumed with a profound sense of inadequacy for being "a high school dropout." Having found her way to where she wanted to be, and feeling happy within herself, she could open her heart to someone else.

In the years since I interviewed Lauren, she has remained happily married and she continues to revel in her role as grandmother. Her stepdaughter is living with Lauren and her husband, along with their granddaughter. Lauren enjoys being able to see them every day. She is also doing well at work. Five years after our interview, she entered a managerial position. She recently told me:

> I sometimes still marvel at the way my life has turned out and take delight in it. I think, "Is this me?" and finally it feels as if it is me. For a long time I didn't think I'd get out of the place where I found myself after the aneurysm. Then, I didn't think I'd really get too far and would long to be somewhere else. I hoped that people didn't think that was where I was, who I was, where I would always be, and I felt like I was a fraud and not very secure as I moved along and maybe couldn't sustain it, and now I feel that yes, this is me, I can do this.

Liz Holtby

BLOODY-MINDED DESPITE IT ALL:

DISEMPOWERMENT AND

DEPRESSION

Liz Holtby had a hemorrhagic stroke in 1970. Like Lauren, she was seventeen. I was able to meet Liz, a woman of Scots and Anglo-Saxon heritage, in person at her home in Scotland in December 2002; she was fifty years old at the time. Her home was undergoing renovations and was not a suitable place to talk, so we conducted the interview at a nearby restaurant.

Liz has had an extremely difficult time coping with the consequences of her stroke. Her life has been filled with anger and depression — emotions that stem from feeling discounted by others. We can also see in Liz's story the significance of support, in this case by looking at the impact of a serious lack of it. Sexuality, motherhood and empowerment also all play an important role.

*

In 1970, Liz was, by her own account, a rebellious teen. She lived with her widowed mother in a small town in northern England and had been working since she was fifteen, first in the uninspiring position of being the "tea girl" in a lawyer's office, and second, working at the telephone exchange — a job that she quite liked. She had left high school at age fourteen and then completed a year of secretarial college. It wasn't the case that the family needed Liz to bring in income. When Liz's father died he had left the family well provided for. Liz simply wanted to start making her own way in the world, but despite having done so, she was unhappy.

To a large extent, Liz's discontent stemmed from her difficult relationship with her mother. Liz found her mother remarkably unaffectionate, unable to show any real emotion. She felt more like a burden to her mother than a cherished daughter. Indeed, Liz cannot recall her mother ever giving her a hug. Thus, she did her best to live outside her mother's purview, and she was even making plans to emigrate to Canada with a friend as soon as she turned eighteen; they had already completed all the necessary paperwork and documentation. As well, she was excited about finally getting her driver's license: she had an appointment scheduled for a test. Things were starting to come together for her.

Liz's driving test was scheduled for a Monday, and the Saturday before, she was making plans to go to a party. She was quite excited about it and had bought a new outfit for the occasion. When she got up that Saturday morning, though, she says:

> I sat down to have some breakfast, and I felt *fine*, and then I took one bite from a piece of toast and pain just shot up the right side of the head. And it just wouldn't go off, it was there, constant, it was just a *throb* all the time. Since then I've had two kids and the pain of that was far worse than childbirth. And then the vision was affected. Then I got sick. So my mom went to the chemist — my vision was like flashing lights, all coloured lights. I couldn't focus on anything, but I was determined that this was going to go off. And I *was* going to wear my new clothes that day. I went and I had a bath, and I don't know how I got in and out of the bath, but after I did, I got dressed in the new clothes and my mother came in and she found me passed out on the bed. Meanwhile the chemist had thought perhaps it was a really bad migraine. My mother came back with something

and she tried to give me something, but I was just vomiting all the time.

That evening, her mother phoned the doctor, who also thought it was a migraine, despite her mother's protests that it was something more. Liz continues:

All through the night I was still vomiting, it was just all bile. There was nothing inside me, it was just pure bile. My mother called the doctor again on Sunday morning and he said, "It's a bad migraine and that's all there is to it." It went on all day, she called the doctor again at night. Now this was a small place so you kind of got put through to the doctor's home. And the doctor's wife answered the phone and she told my mother not to bother her husband on a weekend, it was his day off. And that was all there was to it. Monday morning, she called the surgery [medical clinic], and I'm not sure whether it was the same doctor who came out or a different doctor but, as my mother reminded me many times, within ten *minutes* they had an ambulance at the door. And flashing lights all the way to the hospital.

Liz was taken to the local hospital, which was not large, and was there for about five days while doctors tried to figure out what was wrong with her. As was the case with Lauren Mayes, doctors probably were not very familiar with the signs of hemorrhagic stroke. Liz's head pain became less intense after a few days, but it did not go away completely, and she still wasn't able to see properly. Then she started hearing noises in her ears that sounded like "motorbikes or geese." She recalls that "it was just continuous." On her fifth day there, she was taken in a wheelchair to see the ear, nose and throat specialist, and she recalls feeling very unwell. She remembers that the very movement of the wheelchair caused her head to ache intensely. Then, once she arrived at the room to see the specialist and he started to talk to her, her head went back, her eyes fixed on a light, and she passed out. Liz had just had her first epileptic seizure.

She was immediately transferred to a large neurological centre in Newcastle, where she was bombarded with questions:

One doctor in particular I remember. He asked me, "Do you take drugs?" And then he told my mother, he said, "She must take drugs." He tried this with me so many times, "you *do* take drugs, just admit it. For the sake of your health now, you *have* to admit it." "I don't *take* drugs." "You've never smoked anything, you've never done any drugs?" "No." "Well, what kind of life-style do you lead?" [laugh] It was appalling! It was as if I was on trial! I could hardly see him, I wasn't hearing him properly, and this is *all* I was getting. It got to the point where he was writing things down on a piece of paper: "You must not have heard me properly," and all he could say was, "Do you take drugs?"

After that objectionable interrogation, an angiogram was performed. She was anesthetized for the procedure, and the doctor went in through her jugular vein. The doctor was unable to get conclusive results, though, so the next day he did the procedure again, this time going in through her groin (which is the way the procedure is most commonly done for cases of suspected brain hemorrhage). Even though the procedures were conducted with Liz under anesthetic, she found them most unpleasant because she had always hated being put to sleep.

With the second procedure the doctors found Liz's ruptured AVM, which was the cause of her headaches, vision and hearing problems and her epilepsy. Liz got the news on the day she turned eighteen:

I remember sitting on the ward and my mother had been called in and they told me that there was a cluster of blood vessels on the right side of the brain which had been there, an abnormality, there from birth. And it had taken nearly eighteen years before it leaked. If that was a small leak, I would hope that a big leak would just kill you, because the pain was awful. By that time the pain had stopped, the leak had stopped. And the nurse said, "We now have to arrange for surgery." There was *nothing* about explaining anything, there was no *doctor* there telling me, to tell me exactly what was going on, they wanted me to sign a consent form there and then. And she kept going to my mother: "If it had been yesterday you could have had this signed, but because she's eighteen today and they just dropped the age of majority, it's up to her now." And I wouldn't sign it. I wouldn't sign it and I discharged myself that day.

Presumably, the doctor wanted to surgically remove her AVM, but Liz was never actually told details about the surgery the doctor wanted to perform. It seemed clear to Liz that hospital staff did not consider her entitled to any information about what they were doing or what they thought about her prospects for recovery, and so she rebelled. She refused to sign the consent form for the surgery mostly because of the disrespectful way she had been treated by doctors and nurses ever since her AVM first ruptured. All she knew was that medical professionals who didn't seem to take her seriously were asking her to consent to having her hair shaved off so that her head could be operated on. There was no way she was going to consent to that.

On the one hand, Liz's concern about her appearance can be seen as normal for most teenagers, so it's not surprising that she wouldn't want to have her hair shaved off. This unhappiness about the prospect of having the head shaved was commonly voiced by those women I interviewed who were recommended for brain surgery at any age. No doubt, it is a concern for women particularly, because it is generally considered unacceptable for women to have a shaved head (unlike the case for men). Girls and women learn to value the hair on their heads (but not hair on other body parts), and it is often seen as contributing to women's beauty.

On the other hand, we can see Liz as primarily concerned about being discounted, in that she was expected to simply comply with unexplained dictums, and the fact that staff were preparing to shave her head was the last straw. In this regard, Liz's experience of being ignored might have been precipitated by the fact that she had only that day reached the status of legal adulthood, and so staff were inclined to continue treating her as a child who had no rights. Possibly, her treatment was also a result of her femaleness, and we can speculate that had she been male, she may have been shown more respect. The year, after all, was 1970. While the feminist movement was beginning to re-emerge into the public domain, most people more or less took it for granted that girls and women were not deserving of the same treatment as boys and men.

Liz went home with her mother. As wary as she was of her mother overpowering her, she was frightened by what had happened, her weakness and especially the epileptic seizures, which had become frequent. She felt that it would be safer for her to be with her mother. Her mother, though, wouldn't leave her alone and kept trying to get her to consent to surgery. Before long, Liz had had enough and went to stay with her sister-in-law. But her sister-in-law couldn't cope with Liz's seizures, and Liz had to go back to her mother's house. It began to sink in that an operation could save her, but Liz still would not consider surgery. In her words, "It was like living all the time knowing that you had a time bomb inside your head. And you could just sign the piece of paper and get them to take it away, but, *but* — but I couldn't answer what the 'but' was."

Liz became convinced that the doctors had told her mother that she only had a certain amount of time to live, but when she confronted her mother to ask for the truth, her mother would not say anything. While Liz never did learn exactly what her mother had been told, she was probably told that unless Liz had surgery to remove the AVM it would rupture and cause a massive and lethal brain hemorrhage.

Liz decided that if she had only a limited amount of time to live, she would live as she pleased. She became, she says, even more rebellious than before, although her impairments certainly limited what she could do. She tired very easily so could not exert herself too much without becoming totally drained, and she had extreme right-sided weakness that made many tasks difficult if not impossible to do. But, she explained: "I *hated* the idea of anybody doing anything for me. There was always something inside my head that was saying, 'You can still do this. You might feel weak at the moment but you can still do it.'"

She also had problems with her vision. Most disturbing, though, were the "horrendous" epileptic seizures. In a typical week, she would have three or four "grand mal" seizures. These are the most intense of all types of seizures, and are characterized by a loss of consciousness, body stiffening and shaking, and sometimes tongue biting or loss of bladder control. After the shaking subsides, a period of confusion or sleepiness usually occurs. One week she had these seizures almost daily. Usually, but not always, she would realize that a seizure was about to overtake her because she would suddenly see flashing lights and notice a particular smell, but those were the only warnings Liz had. She learned to recognize what was likely to trigger a seizure, such as bright or flashing lights; discotheques were out. Even bright sunshine could be a problem. Consequently, there were many places that Liz could no longer go. The epilepsy, she said, "caused havoc" in her life. She could cope with the vision problems, she could cope with her right-sided weakness and low level of energy, but she had great difficulty coping with the epilepsy. Not surprisingly, Liz became depressed.

What she *could* do was prove to herself and others that she was an adult woman:

> With me believing that my mother hadn't told me everything, I was determined to prove so much, in such a short space of time. I went out and I lost my virginity, I got pregnant, I got married, and this was just to prove that I could do this. I feel disgusted, actually, when I think about it: just to prove that I could do this, to have a baby. I didn't ever consider for one second that this child may be left without a mother. Do you know, in some ways that's more uncomfortable to talk about than the brain hemorrhage.

At age nineteen, then, Liz married someone related to her sister-in-law whom she had known since childhood. She did not love him — "I didn't really care about this person," she relayed, "I was very selfish at that stage." Liz thinks, meanwhile, that her husband was only interested in her inheritance that her father had placed in trust for her. So, they each used the other for their own purposes.

Pregnancy was not especially difficult for Liz — she doesn't recall that the seizures posed a problem for the pregnancy — but she had to spend the last five weeks in the hospital so that her condition could be closely monitored. No doubt, the doctors were worried that the strain of the pregnancy might cause her AVM to rupture again. When it was time for the delivery, she did not want an epidural because she wanted to experience her labour pains, but doctors were afraid of what would happen if her blood pressure went up, so she was given an epidural anyway — another instance of Liz's wishes being discounted by the medical profession. She was in labour for fifteen hours, and afterwards felt that she had really missed out on something because she had not been able to feel the pains.

Liz had trouble coping with the needs of her new baby daughter. She became even more depressed than before, and frequently felt suicidal. At one point she went so far as to take a knife and cut her wrist. Another time she took a drug overdose. Then, when her baby daughter was nine months old, Liz had had enough of her loveless marriage to a husband who drank a lot. She took her baby daughter, walked out and went back to her mother. Although she had succeeded in proving that she could marry and have a child, it clearly was not a route to happiness. Quite the contrary, the marriage was, in Liz's words, "a total sham and never really stood a chance."

A few years later Liz decided that her daughter needed a sibling, so she entered into a casual liaison with her former husband and got pregnant again. Once again, she was given an epidural for the delivery, but this time the epidural did not work so effectively and Liz was able to experience her labour pains. Her second daughter was born three years after her first.

Liz was only able to cope with being a mother because she was living with her own mother who helped considerably with caring for the children. Liz loved her daughters and did not hesitate to express her affection, so that they would not grow up feeling unloved as she had. Yet she remained depressed. She took anti-depressive medication off and on, but it did not seem to help. She also took anti-seizure medication, but this did not seem to prevent her from having violent seizures. For years, she existed in this depressed state.

If, within the first few years after her stroke, anyone had asked her to talk about how she felt or shown an interest in listening to her, things might have turned out very differently. But after years of being ignored, she gave up hope that anyone cared about how she had been affected. Her suicide attempts were not so much serious attempts to end her own life as they were cries for help and understanding. Still, her cries went unanswered. Certainly her mother, helpful as she was with raising Liz's children, was no more prepared than she had ever been to listen with loving attention to what Liz had to say. There was no one who seemed willing to help Liz work through her thoughts and feelings about all that had happened to her. By the time she was twenty-one, she had closed the door to her feelings so that, even if someone had offered to talk to her with compassion, she doubts that she would have opened up.

> No one had listened to me. I was just being told, "Do this, do that, you shouldn't be doing this, take this and take that." "Why?" "Because that's what we've prescribed." "Yes, but why?" And I got to the point where I didn't even ask why. Because I just knew that I wasn't going to be answered and it was not going to come.

Things began to change when, at age thirty, Liz fell down the stairs as a result of an epileptic seizure, injuring her foot. She went to hospital to have it seen to, and while there, she was also seen by a neurologist who talked her into having another angiogram done to check on her AVM. The test results showed that the AVM was growing and getting ready to burst. The doctor scared Liz when he told her that when it burst — not if, but when — she would not be as lucky as the last time. It was highly unlikely that she would survive a second bleed.

Unlike her initial physicians, Liz felt that this doctor treated her with respect. He didn't judge her or accuse her of doing anything wrong. Rather, he sat down with her and carefully explained everything he could. Liz listened closely to what he had to say. The doctor told her that he might be able to surgically remove the AVM before it burst, but he couldn't guarantee the success of the operation. He also told her that, because the AVM was very close to her optic nerve, there was the possibility of her right eye becoming damaged and she could even become blind in that eye. He asked her to think about going ahead with the surgery, and he asked her to consider her two young children as she decided what to do.

Liz quickly came to the conclusion that, because of her children, she didn't have a choice but to go through with the surgery. The respect the doctor had shown was also a major factor in her decision to go ahead. As frightening as the prospect of brain surgery was to Liz, she nevertheless felt empowered by finally being able to give her informed consent. She agreed to undergo the surgery and it was scheduled for February 1983.

Once she decided to have the surgery, she set about preparing her daughters, then aged eleven and eight. Fortunately, there was a timely television program on brain surgery that they were all able to watch together. Her youngest daughter cried all through the program, but Liz was adamant that her children be informed about what was going to happen. She had arguments with her mother about this, but Liz did not want them feeling left out. Her insistence that they be included in everything was rooted in her own memories of being sent away for six weeks when her father died. No one ever discussed his death with her, and Liz had felt pushed away. Her mother acquiesced. Indeed, after the surgery she brought them to see Liz, going so far as to argue with the hospital staff who did not want to let the children into the room.

Liz's long hair was shaved off for the surgery. The surgery lasted ten and a half hours, and was videotaped to be used for teaching purposes. Liz is fascinated to know that a videotape exists, although she has never been offered the opportunity to watch it. After the surgery, she was impressed that her doctors came to sit with her and told her everything she wanted to know about how the operation went. They told her that it was a great success and that her AVM was permanently removed. She could rest assured that she was not at risk of having it grow again or burst. Her eyesight was also saved, although her right eye has been noticeably weak ever since. As well, she periodically experiences "visual disturbances," exacerbated by bright sunlight or strobe lighting. The biggest bonus, following the surgery, was that she never again had a "grand mal" seizure; however, they were replaced with "petit mal" seizures. Luckily she finds these relatively easy to cope with, as they consist mostly of simply "blanking out" for a few seconds.

Liz is convinced that if she had agreed to the surgery when she was eighteen, it would not have been the success it was when she was thirty. She believes that she had two far better surgeons the second time around.

Liz has also taken control of when and how much of her anti-seizure medication she takes. She decided on her own to start reducing the dosage before gaining her doctor's approval, and in recent years, she has almost stopped taking anti-seizure medication altogether. She never wants to be without the medication, however, as she will still take it on the days when she feels especially vulnerable to a seizure. Her doctor tells her that the medication doesn't work this way, that in order to have it prevent a seizure it is necessary to take it continuously, but Liz is convinced that, at least in her case, taking her anti-seizure tablets only when she feels vulnerable does work to prevent a seizure. In this regard, Liz is taking control of her own medical care — something that she was unable to do when younger. Her newfound ability to monitor her own medical needs is empowering, and sharply contrasts with her early experiences of powerlessness.

There have been disasters as a result of a "petit mal" seizure. Once she "blanked out" and fell down the stairs. Fortunately, nothing serious happened, but she was taken to the hospital and had yet another angiogram, which showed nothing untoward to be concerned about. Another time she momentarily lost consciousness as she was crossing the road. She stepped into the road only to be hit by the side of a bus and she was thrown to the pavement. The bus driver stopped and ran over to her with great concern. He wanted to call an ambulance for Liz, but Liz would not let him. She had suffered a badly bruised arm, but other than that only her pride was hurt. There was no way she was going to let anyone take her to the hospital. She had come to hate the very smell of hospitals.

With a new lease on life, Liz decided to move away from her mother. She left the English town where she had always lived and moved to Scotland, where she had an aunt with whom she enjoyed being. Then, when her oldest daughter was studying for her school "O" level examinations, Liz realized that she would like to go back to school herself. She especially enjoyed studying history, so she enrolled in a pre-university course. Her neurologists, meanwhile, advised her not to even try going to school, telling her that her memory had been impaired and she would never be able to cope with trying to remember a great deal of information. But Liz had had enough of others telling her what she could or could not do:

> All the time, the neurologists were saying, "You will never be able to do this, you will never be able to do that, your memory will never hold this." And I thought, "You swines I'll prove you *wrong*!" Again, bloody-minded, and I *was* determined to prove them wrong, I got top marks. The next year I did higher history. And I got an A. Um, top marks again. The year after that I went in to do — what was it I did? What they call Modern Studies here, it's sociology and politics. I got B for that. What else — and I did English literature, grammar and I got an A for that. The following year, I did anatomy, physiology and health and I got a B for that. And then I went to university.

At the university level, though, Liz had trouble coping with the work, and she had to give it up. She suspects that the problem was not that the work really was too difficult for her. She thinks she could have coped with the assignments had she not had to worry about finances and work at the same time.

After a few years, Liz began to regret that she hadn't persevered in her university education. One day, however, Liz was telling someone about her interest in midwifery, and her friend suggested that she ought to go into the profession. In her forties, then, Liz decided to apprentice to become a midwife. It was a remarkable decision, given her dislike of hospitals (in the UK, midwives are commonly present for hospitals births), but Liz absolutely loved it. Her "petit mal" seizures were more or less under control with medication and not really disabling. Nor did she experience her right-sided weakness as significantly disabling. Like so many of us who have one-sided weakness, she had early on in her post-stroke life learned to compensate, so that others rarely even noticed that there was any difficulty with things requiring fine motor skills.

Nevertheless, Liz was not happy with her mentor, who was in her opinion judgemental and uncaring. The last straw for Liz was when her mentor chastised her for being nice to a seventeen-year-old who was delivering her second child. Her mentor, according to Liz, did not think the young mother was deserving of any respect. Liz told her mentor that she was glad she didn't have a midwife like her when she was delivering her own children. Liz, no doubt, was remembering what it was like herself when she was eighteen years old and no one seemed to want to show her any respect. Perhaps also, though Liz did not say this, she was drawn to midwifery in the first place because she felt very strongly that a woman ought to be able to control the birthing process, and so becoming a midwife represented an opportunity to help women have a better childbirth experience than she herself had experienced.

After that incident, Liz did not continue her training. She had begun taking care of her mother who had become ill and financial circumstances continued to be difficult. Just as with her attempt to go to university, Liz once again found that she had to give up a dream.

Although Liz had never had a good relationship with her mother, she always remained in close contact with her. So, when Liz began to hear her mother saying strange things on the telephone, she went to investigate what was going on. She found her mother doing things such as putting an electric kettle on the gas stove, and realized that her mother, who was now in her eighties, was becoming senile. At that point, she brought her mother to live with her. Liz's mother has become progressively sicker since moving in with her. On top of worsening dementia, four years after moving in her mother went into heart failure. She was hospitalized and given two months to live. Liz insisted she come home; she didn't want her mother dying in hospital or in a home.

Three years later, Liz was still caring for her mother at home. Doctors, who had been so sure that she would not live much longer, were amazed. All they could say was that Liz must be taking very good care of her. Liz is a very caring and compassionate woman, but she often finds it a strain to be the sole caregiver, especially because she has developed arthritis in her hands, continues to have right-sided weakness and, since her stroke, has always tired easily. Fatigue is one of those invisible impairments that can be particularly disabling, because it is such a subjective feeling. There are rarely any visible clues to tell an onlooker that one is feeling too fatigued to carry on with an activity. Indeed, we stroke survivors often have trouble ourselves recognizing that we are getting tired and it would be a good idea to take a rest. Typically, we carry on until suddenly it is no longer possible to carry on. Everything becomes a challenge when feeling stroke-related fatigue, and it can be particularly galling to have someone tell us that we simply need to push through it.

In any case, Liz's impairments are not as easy to deal with now that she is in her fifties. She is generally able to enjoy being with her mother. She suspects that this may be because she is now the one in charge of the situation; her mother is no longer able to dominate her. In any case, from time to time Liz will give her mother a cuddle, and they frequently laugh and joke together. At other times, though not very often, Liz can be "very bad tempered with her." When this happens, she finds it's best to just walk away from the situation. Liz says that "there are still days when I resent it," especially because it is so physically taxing for her. She sometimes gets quite depressed about the situation.

Every so often, one of Liz's daughters will come for a few weeks so that Liz can take a vacation. They are the only ones who offer Liz any relief. Certainly Liz's stepbrother — from her mother's first marriage and fourteen years her senior — has not offered to help with caring for their mother. Liz has never, in any case, been on good terms with him. When she was a child, she idolized him but he regarded her as "just the pest of a kid sister." He showed more interest in Liz when she was about to inherit her father's small legacy, but when she would not let him have any of her money, he went back to paying no attention to her. He seemed to show little interest in their mother as well. In fact, there was a two-year period after their mother went into heart failure when he did not even call to see how she was doing.

In considering Liz's life after her stroke, it would have been nice if, after she had her AVM surgically removed at age thirty and there was no longer anything to cause a full-blown epileptic seizure, she had been able to reinvent herself and emerge a new woman. She did, after all, have two young daughters who loved her and whom she loved in return. Yet such a fairy tale plot does not do justice to the complexity of life. By age thirty, Liz had spent almost half her life — certainly all of her adult life — never knowing when she would experience a "grand mal" epileptic seizure. She had been forced to organize her life so that she would not be in situations that she knew would produce a seizure. She was fearful of living alone. She was, moreover, always mindful that her AVM represented a time-bomb inside her head: it could go off at any time. Just getting through a day without mishap could be a struggle, and it's not surprising that Liz lived with deep depression. So, by the time the threat of a full-blown seizure was removed from her life at age thirty, she had few resources that would allow her to take stock of her life and make radical changes. Her doctors continued to reinforce that she had permanent impairments that would prevent her from accomplishing many things that she might otherwise want to do.

For all these reasons, even after her surgery, Liz remained mostly depressed for the next fifteen years or so. Depression is something Liz is intimately familiar with. When she stands back to analyze where her depression comes from, she thinks that it stems from a lifetime of feeling that no one wanted to listen to her or treat her with respect. Starting with her mother when she was a child, she was continually told what to do with no explanation. As she said, "My mother never tried to talk me into anything, my mother tried to dictate." Although she later took tentative steps towards changing her life — arguably the most significant step being the move away from her mother — more often than not, circumstances intervened to thwart whatever plans she might have. Ever since her stroke at age seventeen, this seemed to be the story of her life.

Had Liz felt that others cared about her feelings, she might not have sunk ever deeper into depression as the years wore on. As it was, all she ever heard were admonishments about what she could *not* do. No one seemed interested in exploring, let alone celebrating, what she *could* do. No one talked about her strengths — just her weaknesses and shortcomings. She explains:

> I still can get depressed, but I don't — I kind of have a different way of dealing with it now. When I first came to Scotland, I had no confidence, I had so many doctors telling me: "You'll never be able to this, you'll never be able to do that. You'll never — don't even think about doing that because your memory has been affected, and you will never be able to — don't even entertain the idea of such and such," whatever it was. And *that* used to depress me so much. It all lifted when I knew that I *could* do things. And that doctors were *not* always right. At first, because I was feeling really quite weak and quite down, I think there was a kind of acceptance of what they were saying. I thought, "Oh well that's it." But I started to read a lot and I thought, "No, no, no, you're not right! I'm not taking notice of everything you say!" They — a lot of them go by the book and this is what the book says and that's it. It doesn't work like that.

Although Liz has done relatively well since her surgery at age thirty, her emotions surrounding her stroke-related experiences are raw, and she remains bitter. She said that "in the end the outcome was positive, but over the years there was so much depression." Beyond recognizing that she had beat the odds in that many people who have a brain hemorrhage do not live, she was not philosophical about anything that had happened. Indeed, barely a day goes by without her being reminded of how her life was irretrievably changed: "It's *dictated* everything that I've been able to *do*. Any pain in the head, any headache and I *still* to this day panic. I can tell you every *detail* of that day [that it happened]. That never left me. Never."

It was only when she happened, by chance, to come across my request for survivors' stories, that she began to entertain the thought of telling someone about what happened. She said:

> I kind of looked at it and thought, "Oh god, there's a bad memory!" I guess I was curious as to what you wanted to know. It's strange, I don't think I've ever sat and talked about this to anybody like this! I think I just reached a stage in life where it was — I had to talk about this. Because it's still there, you know?

*

In part, Liz has spent her life not talking about the momentous event of her stroke and the aftermath because no one ever asked. Another possibly more important reason, though, is that there is little space in everyday life for an understanding of the experiences of those of us who have survived a life-threatening event such as hemorrhagic stroke. Particularly in a post-industrial society that goes to great lengths to deny the frailty of the human body, it is difficult to talk about that frailty and what it can feel like. For those of us, like Liz, who at first glance appear to be able-bodied, we are expected to *be* able-bodied. Indeed, to a large extent we learn — even if we can't articulate it as such — that we are acceptable in mainstream society only to the extent that we don't upset the expectations of others, including the expectation that we have never faced a life-threatening trauma and we are as fully capable as we appear. In the face of these social expectations, and especially considering that she felt discounted, how *could* Liz have talked about her experiences? It seems obvious that, to preserve her own sense of self-respect, she could not broach the topic of her stroke and its consequences. In many ways, it was easier for her to go through life, as it is easier for so many of us in similar circumstances, pretending that she was no different from anyone else.

When things cannot be hidden, we typically hide from others, rather than have them see what is, in a very real sense, *unspeakable*. For Liz, this meant a lifetime of internalizing her anger.

Finally, Liz's experiences are, in a larger sense, quintessentially a woman's experiences. Men, of course, can get seriously depressed, but statistics tell us that women are far more likely to internalize their anger, to pretend that everything is okay when it is not and, as a result, to become hopelessly depressed. We women are expected to be the caregivers in society — Liz's life shows what can happen when there is no one to take care of the caregiver. It is a testament to Liz's strength of character that she has managed to accomplish so much — such as lovingly raise two daughters, go back to school and care for her mother — and remain on an even keel.

Esther Stein

RE-IMAGINING ONESELF:

SELF-IMAGE AND ABUSE

Esther Stein's story has a special significance for me, as it was Esther's article I had found in the journal that day in the library. She was twenty-four when her AVM ruptured in 1982. Esther had written mostly about what it was like to be a patient in the hospital, and she wrote in great detail about what she felt and thought about what was going on around her. Her account not only brought up a lot of memories for me, it also served as an affirmation of my own experience. In an important sense, Esther was the inspiration for embarking on my project of collecting the narratives of young women stroke survivors. I doubt I ever would have begun it had I not first known of Esther's existence.

I didn't get to meet Esther face to face until a blustery Sunday afternoon in March of 2001, when I made my way to her home in Buffalo, New York. Esther, who is Jewish, was forty-three at the time. Since she had already written about her hospitalization experiences, we focused on talking about what happened afterwards, and why she thought things turned out as they have. When I later reflected on what she had told me, I began to see that an important aspect of her experiences can be understood in terms of self-image and abuse. Her self-image suffered terribly as a result of the stroke, and this made her vulnerable to psychological abuse by her partner. Like Liz Holtby's, Esther's is very much a woman's story.

Other themes reflected in Esther's story revolve around motherhood, romantic relationships and financial resources. In telling her story, I draw in part on what she told me when we met and in part on her written account.

*

In 1982, Esther Stein was an attractive and academically gifted young woman, and for these reasons she felt special. As the youngest of three girls in her family, she had grown into adulthood with an urge to prove herself capable of independence. Secretly, she cherished a sense of superiority. She had, after all, been accepted into university at the age of seventeen, and by twenty, she was starting graduate school. She had a quick mind and could talk circles around anyone who cared to debate her. At twenty-three, she graduated with a master's degree in library science. A few months later, she was working as an assistant librarian at a small public library in Buffalo, and she was wondering what it would be like to become the chief librarian at a more prestigious institution. At the same time, she was still not entirely sure that she really wanted to remain in the field. Although she liked the work, she had felt pressured by her parents to choose library science over becoming a historian, which was what she really found fascinating. While she took great pride in her professional achievements, she was feeling a sense of unease over what she would do in terms of her career.

She was also going through rough times in her personal life. In November 1981, only a few months after she had started her job as a librarian, her father became extremely ill and deteriorated rapidly. He died in February 1982:

> I had been very close to him, I was really devastated. It was the first major loss of my life. I had had grandparents who died but you know this was — he was not old, he was sixty-three, and

he went from perfect health to death within months. All we knew was that he had a strange illness. In retrospect — this is a whole other story — it appears he had AIDS. This was the very beginning of the epidemic, so we didn't know that at the time. He just died very rapidly. I was … it was such a shock and such a loss, I didn't know what had hit me. And so, at the time immediately leading up to the stroke, I wasn't that focused on my career anymore. It was like, I had this exciting job and I was excited to be a young professional and I was thinking of doing something different. But then I had this tremendous loss in my life.

As well, Esther was living with her boyfriend, Simon, but the relationship was not going well. Simon had a bad temper, and he had been particularly unsympathetic when Esther's father became ill and died. Esther may not have labelled him abusive at the time, but she was clear that she didn't want to be with him any longer. She was preparing to break up with him.

On July 2, 1982, Esther's day began much as any other, although when she woke up she felt a little nauseated and there was a faint buzzing in her head. She did her best to ignore her subtle feelings of unwellness and went to work. The morning passed uneventfully and then it was time for lunch with a friend. The buzzing in her head was still there and even becoming a little worse, but Esther put it down to anxiety. As she went off to lunch, things became critical:

I was vaguely aware that something odd was going on. I could not walk straight and bumped into columns and walls on my left side. My friend was very concerned but I insisted that I was just tired. At lunch, unable to balance on the chair, I listed to the left. Food dribbled out of the left side of my mouth. As we headed back to our office, I stumbled. Ignoring my protests, my friend called out "She needs an ambulance." Two good Samaritans picked me up (I am quite small: 5 feet 2 inches, 110 lbs.) and put me on the floor of the nearest building. I was surprised that even lying down the spinning in my head did not stop. The last thing I remembered from that strange day was breathing through an oxygen mask in the ambulance. I am told that I was first taken to a local hospital where the diagnosis of stroke was made, and then sent to the excellent neurological intensive care unit at a larger hospital.

Five days later, Esther woke up from a coma to find herself in the hospital's intensive care unit (ICU). She recognized where she was as soon as she woke up — she had become all too familiar with the sights and sounds after spending so much time with her father in ICU before he died. She assumed that because she was in ICU, she too was going to die, and so she tried to remember the words to "Hear, O Israel," the prayer traditionally said by Jews before death. Then familiar faces appeared at her bedside.

Her boyfriend, Simon, and her sister, Ellen, filled her in on what had happened. They assured her that she was not going to die. She had had a brain hemorrhage, they said, due to a ruptured AVM. This had been diagnosed not long after she arrived at the first hospital, where she had been given a CT scan and an angiogram. Esther was so relieved to learn that she wasn't dying that she did not at first stop to consider the significance of what she was being told. She soon drifted back into unconsciousness.

Over the next few days, she would go back and forth between consciousness and unconsciousness, not really aware that her entire left side was paralyzed. Esther recalls an experience that was almost exactly the same as one that Lauren Mayes had while hospitalized — she woke up to find herself holding someone's hand, but when she looked around to see who it was, there was no one there. Only then did she realize that she was holding her own left hand. Before she had time to ponder what this meant, her mother appeared and told her that she had had a stroke. This confused Esther because the only thing she knew about stroke was that her grandfather had had one at the age of eighty.

Gradually, as Esther spent more and more time awake, she became aware of how uncomfortable she was feeling. She had a tube in each arm and one in her nose and down her throat so that liquids could be fed into her stomach. Small black sticky patches attached wires from her chest to a machine, and she had a catheter that she found extremely itchy. It was a relief, then, when doctors deemed her stable enough to be disconnected from the various tubes and wires and moved to a semi-private room.

By this time, she was vaguely aware of what had happened to her, but she was still confused about what it all meant. At first, she was mostly content to accept the congratulations that visitors proffered because she had survived a potentially fatal event. After a while, though, it dawned on Esther that the visitors who were congratulating her on her luck in surviving were walking around, while she lay in bed with the entire left side of her body paralyzed. She later wrote:

> With my left side completely paralyzed, I was as helpless as a fish on land. I couldn't dress myself, eat, sit up or urinate without assistance. This condition was humiliating. I couldn't get used to performing toilet functions in public on a bedpan. I felt like I was being toilet trained all over again; if I was a good girl and "produced," a woman would coo "go-oo-od." My total helplessness, the sensation of being cared for and the involvement of various women in my every intimate function simulated a return to babyhood.

It was when she began physical therapy that Esther began starting to appreciate just how much work she would have to do in order to recover. The first thing she had to do was get used to sitting up for extended periods, but that was easier said than done. She was amazed to find that she would become dizzy after only about thirty seconds, and she had to work her way up to sitting for more than a few hours. She had to get used to using a wheelchair for transportation to therapy, which she found terrifying because she had never sat in a wheelchair before. In physical therapy, she had to get used to lying helplessly on a mat while the therapist "ranged" (moved around) her left arm and leg to prevent them from stiffening. Then the therapist put a metal brace on her left leg from her ankle to her hip, and asked her to try taking a few steps. Esther held on to her therapist's neck to take a few shaky steps, and fearfully wondered if she would ever again walk normally.

Occupational therapy was also a shock for Esther. The occupational therapist explained that she would help her adapt to her disability, but Esther didn't want to have to adapt. She was expecting a full recovery of her pre-stroke abilities. She shook with horror over learning that, even if she did make a full recovery, it would not be for a very long time. Reluctantly, she began learning how to operate a wheelchair and she practised ways of getting up and down from a sitting position.

The strangest experience for Esther was speech therapy, but it was also extremely important for her self-esteem. She had been proud of her facility with spoken language and was horrified to find that she had trouble making herself understood because of slurred and indistinct speech. She couldn't control the intonation in her voice, so that even when her words were clearly spoken, her intent was often misunderstood. Equally distressing, she explains, were that the muscles on the left side of her face were so slack that her smile seemed to be "up somewhere near her right ear." She would look in the mirror as she practised making sounds and wonder who the strange looking person was who couldn't talk right. She practised her mouth exercises diligently, desperately wanting to regain at least her speech as quickly as she could.

After a month at the acute-care hospital, her doctors agreed that she had recovered sufficiently to be moved to a rehabilitation facility. Her mother found a facility with a good reputation that also had a bed available immediately. Esther was excited about the move as she equated it with recovery. The Gibson Center, which Esther's mother had described to her in glowing terms, was outside of the city. Esther began imagining a stay there, in a lovely collegiate setting, as a kind of vacation. She imagined herself strolling around the grounds. She pictured herself at the mirror fixing her hair before having dinner with handsome male patients.

The reality of the Gibson Center was quite different, and Esther was bitterly disappointed when she got there to find that it was simply another hospital:

> My room was on a floor with other young spinal and brain
> trauma patients, mostly young men injured in motorcycle, car
> and swimming accidents, including several young quadriple-

gics. The majority of the patients, however, were elderly stroke and cardiac patients. There were no other young stroke patients and I felt as if, by some bizarre time warp, I had suddenly become elderly and ended up in a nursing home at twenty-four. In the first few days at Gibson I came face to face with my physical and social helplessness in a way that I had not previously done.

She sank into depression and anger. She felt that "life was tremendously unfair, capricious and cruel. I couldn't believe that this rare and freakish catastrophe had hit me only five months after the terrible blow of the equally freakish death of my adored father."

She even considered suicide, and spent time fantasizing about how she would do it, given her physical limitations. It was only after Simon pointed out to her that if she tried to get better she might recover, but if she gave up she would surely lose, that she began to see that she needed to focus on recovering as much as possible.

Simon's support was invaluable to her during her hospitalization. He came to see her every day and spent hours with her, holding her, washing and dressing her, and helping her with toileting. Her thoughts about breaking up with him were forgotten: "At the risk of extreme sentimentality, I must comment on the sustaining power of love. His empathy with the most minute details of living with the paralysis greatly diminished my isolation."

At the Gibson Center, Esther spent a lot of time in physical therapy, working to regain as much use of her left side as possible. As she was able to see her own progress, her mood improved. She also learned how to do "activities of daily living" with one hand, such as how to dress herself or tie her shoes. About this, she wrote:

Early one morning, Karen, my occupational therapist, arrived to teach me how to dress myself with one hand, an incredibly difficult undertaking. Following her instructions, I practised placing my limp left arm into a rolled up sleeve. Inevitably, when I got my right arm into the other sleeve my left arm flopped out. Deeply embarrassed, I eventually succeeded by moving very slowly and carefully in getting both arms in the sleeves at once. With a sigh of relief, I wriggled into a very twisted T-shirt. (Learning to put on a bra with one hand was so complicated that I will not even attempt to describe it.) At last, using one lace and making a sort of slip-knot with one hand she showed me a method of lacing my sneakers. I remembered the feeling of triumph the first time, twenty years before, that I had tied my very own shoes. I felt humiliated to be learning again at age twenty-four, how to tie my shoes and dress myself. Nothing that I had studied or attempted in the intervening twenty years was as hard as relearning how to dress.

After Esther had been at Gibson for almost two months, she became anxious to go home. She had, by then, recovered her ability to speak clearly, and she had progressed from using a wheelchair to using a cane. Her doctors thought she should stay at Gibson for another few months, but Esther felt she would make better progress away from the institution. The memory of her father's dehumanizing hospital stay and death earlier that year was fresh in her mind. She railed against her own dehumanization, at "the experience of being dressed and shuttled around like an inanimate object on wheels. This desire to assert my humanity now motivated me to leave the protected environment of Gibson as soon as I could dress myself and go to the toilet."

Shortly before Esther left Gibson for good, she was allowed to go on a day trip to her mother's apartment. As she left the hospital grounds, she felt "an enormous sense of exhilaration and freedom," and she was reminded of the last line from *One Flew Over the Cuckoo's Nest*, in which a man escapes institutionalization: "I been away a long time."

In late September, almost three months after her stroke, Esther's mother helped her make her own final escape from institutionalization. At first she moved in with her mother and sister, but a short time later she moved back in with Simon. She was not walking well, but with the help of a cane, at least she was walking. She got rid of her leg brace, even though it gave her stability; it was uncomfortable and offended her vanity ("I'm very vain about my appearance," she told me). In retrospect, she said that she wishes she'd worn it longer, as she might have been able to avert the problems she has now with her ankle and knee. Her knee has become particularly troublesome, as she has developed arthritis, which can be quite painful at times. Her doctor tells her that it was caused by the way that she walks.

When Esther arrived back home, she could not use her left arm. It hung limply at her side, but she maintained hope that with time and effort, she would regain that too. She wasted no time in arranging to become an out-patient at a rehab centre near her home, and she started to take an active interest in her treatment. She began to realize that she might never recover fully, but there were still a lot of things that she *could* do. As well, there was the hope that if she worked at it hard enough and long enough, she would improve over time. This hope kept Esther going regularly for physical therapy for almost four years, mostly paid for with the medical insurance she had from her employer. After that, she reached a plateau where she was unable to notice new improvements and stopped going. The expense was also a factor in her decision to stop, as her insurance would only partially cover the sessions.

In retrospect, Esther said that she thought she gave up on physical therapy too soon; that if she had stuck with it, she would have continued to improve in terms of functional ability. She acknowledged that she could be very critical of herself, and she sometimes felt that she should be doing more than she was to keep her body in good shape. From a different perspective, though, we can see that Esther actually persevered with therapy for a much longer time than many other women. In part, she was able to do this because she had comprehensive medical insurance, but even that policy was not so generous that all of her rehabilitation therapy was covered. Moreover, it was not always easy to get the partial reimbursement that she was entitled to under the terms of the policy. In this regard, her ability to understand legalities and argue her case has served her well. She wondered, though, how others who had less understanding of legalities managed to receive payments from insurance companies.

As it was, a few years after she gave up on physical therapy she started going to a Chinese acupuncturist for treatments. Due to atrophied muscles in her arm and leg, Esther had trouble holding herself completely upright. The acupuncturist was able to help her straighten her body, which made a tremendous difference in her ability to walk and feel better about herself. She stopped going for treatments after about six months — he had begun to molest her during treatments. Esther said: "He was supposed to be working under my arm and he's fondling my breast, and I tried to get him to stop but he pretended not to understand English. But I know he understood that it was a problem."

We can't know whether the acupuncturist molested all of his female patients, but it is significant that women who are especially vulnerable, such as girls and disabled women, are more likely than others to be sexually abused. Given Esther's impairments, he probably did not expect that she would resist. Yet she did resist, and ultimately she used her power to end treatment. She was fortunate that she was in a position to stop going. So often, disabled women are not able to put a stop to sexual abuse, either because they are physically incapable of resisting or because their caregivers do not believe them when they say they are being molested.

In the first year following her return home, Esther worked to reintegrate herself into some semblance of ordinary life. She wrote:

> I found that doing even simple tasks required a great deal of time, patience and ingenuity. However, mastering small household tasks gave me the confidence to venture outside. The first time I did the grocery shopping was a triumph. Negotiating the narrow aisles of a supermarket while trying to steer a full shopping cart with one hand was a nightmare. Part of the problem came from the fact that my arm was not obviously incapacitated, and people in the market looked at me angrily, not really understanding why this young woman was letting her shopping cart waver all over the aisles. In response to their protests I could have said, "I can't move this shopping cart; I have a paralyzed arm." But to preserve my privacy, I remained grimly silent for such an announcement would trigger the inevitable inquiry:

"What happened to you?" "I had a stroke," I reply. "But you are so young! How old are you?" "I am twenty-five now, but I was twenty-four when it happened." Astonished gasp. The stunned silence is long and awkward. I smile cheerfully, shrug and move on. I am used to this routine. Seeing a young person limping, with one arm hanging and no visible marks, makes people understandably curious. The most absurd thing is that most people are so unprepared for the shocking explanation elicited by their nosiness.

Esther returned to work after spending close to a year at home. But looking back, she feels she should have given herself more time. She had been nervous, however, that they wouldn't hold her job.

From the moment Simon learned of Esther's stroke he was there for her, a constant and reassuring presence. Esther felt that she couldn't have had a more loyal friend. While still in the hospital, she had begun to focus on all that was wonderful about him, and she dismissed her earlier misgivings about continuing the relationship. After she returned home to live with him again, she found that he was just as loving and considerate. She felt more comfortable turning to him for help than to her mother or sister.

She felt immense gratitude towards him, and that blossomed into love. She felt that Simon understood her and she could imagine going through the rest of her life with him. A year after she had been home again, she and Simon got married. It was, for Esther, "an occasion of unsurpassed joyousness."

Esther's joy was only compounded a year after her marriage, when she gave birth to her first child, Lisa. She said:

> I always wanted children. That's what I wanted more than anything. Also at the time we were getting involved in traditional Judaism and being fruitful and multiplying is like a core tradition of Judaism. We were around people who were having babies and when I held a baby in my lap I had a supercharged hormonal reaction — I've got to have one. I was really scared shitless, it was very hard. I had a physical therapist at the time who said she believed that I could have children. And then this physical therapist put me in touch with another physical thera-

pist who had just had a baby and she took me on as a private client and she let me handle the baby. It was just amazing that she did that for me. I was very scared. She had a nice, placid baby who was co-operative in the endeavour, so we practised with me holding the baby. And you know of everything I've done, having children was the hardest.

Pregnancy was physically hard on Esther because her swollen belly meant that her centre of gravity was thrown off. It was hard enough walking at the best of times, but like most of us who live with hemiplegia, she had learned how to move her body to compensate for her one-sided weakness. Pregnancy, however, meant that her body changed continually, and she did not always know how to move without mishap. She fell three times while pregnant.

Giving birth was also hard, because her doctor insisted that she have a Caesarean birth, and it took her months to recover from the surgery. At the time, she was willing to take her doctor's advice without questioning his reasoning too closely, but with the passage of time she has gained more knowledge, and has come to realize that many women are forced by their doctors to have a Caesarean section when there really aren't good medical justifications. As Esther said at the time of the interview:

> I think it was a ridiculous thing that I had to have a Caesarean the first time. I think that the obstetrician was the kind of un-scrupulous doctor who — a Caesarean takes half an hour and they make three thousand dollars, a vaginal delivery might take twenty-four hours and they get a thousand dollars, so I think he was unscrupulous, or he was insulating himself from any liability. You know, it was defensive medicine. I don't think it was medically necessary.

Then, coping with her "super-lively animated baby" was almost more than Esther could do. She said, "She would have been a challenging child for any mother, but she was really hard for me." She thinks she was only able to manage mothering a baby who was constantly flailing about because of all the help she had. Most important, Simon spent a lot of time caring for Lisa.

Three months after Lisa's birth, feeling overwhelmed both physically and emotionally, Esther went back to work. She and Simon didn't need the extra income that Esther could earn, but she felt pressured by Simon to return. He told her that she shouldn't be sitting at home doing nothing. Esther didn't agree that she was sitting around doing nothing — it took all the energy she had to care for herself, her baby and her home. But she went along with what he said, in part because she remained so dependent on him to help her with doing so many things that most people take for granted. As well, she continued to feel a sense of gratitude towards Simon because he was so willing to help her with things society deemed her responsibility, such as home and baby.

As Lisa grew, behaviours that had been evident in Simon before marriage began to slowly reappear. Esther describes the way Simon almost seemed to relish her physical weakness, which she surmises was because it gave him the opportunity to take control. The stronger she became both physically and emotionally, the more Simon seemed to want to dominate her. He was able to do it, moreover, because Esther's sense of self-esteem had suffered terribly as a result of the stroke. In her marriage, she felt weak, powerless, inferior. Inside herself, she wasn't sure that she deserved better treatment:

> He never would tell me that I was attractive or compliment me. So, you know, my insecurity was that I had lost my physical attractiveness in the world, and it wasn't objectively true but that was my fear and he manipulatively played upon it. And he had to do a lot with the baby, I mean much more than most men. And he did it, but he wouldn't do it with grace. He did it, but he was very demeaning to me. I would feel that I was sort of — I didn't count, this was his baby and I had just sort of been the womb. He did everything for the baby 'cause I couldn't. We'd go for a walk and, um, he would take the baby stroller and he would march down the street a block ahead of me, and I couldn't keep up, and I'd say, "I want to walk together with you," and he's like, "I can't walk that slow."

By the time Lisa was three, Esther "had something close to a nervous breakdown." She ended up quitting her job to stay home with Lisa, which helped her to feel better about herself, and "it took some of the pressure off the marriage." Esther was now able to focus her energy on taking care of herself, her family and her home, rather than deplete her limited energy reserves outside the home during the day.

Staying home with Lisa, though, could be quite a struggle for Esther. Esther told the following story:

> She used to have tantrums. She would scream and her eyes would roll back in her head. She was so strong-willed that *nothing*, nothing could get through to her. One time, I'd taken her for a walk and it was very cold. We got to the store and she wanted to buy ice cream at the store and eat it outside on the steps, because that's what we did in summer. I said no, and she stood outside the store and screamed. I couldn't *physically* pick her up and drag her home, which is what another mother could do. Oh, I remember this so vividly! And I thought, well, we can't stand here, it's freezing, it's getting dark. I'm going to start walking away.
>
> You're not supposed to threaten children with abandonment in the first place, but I had no choice. Most children would have been: "Mommy! Mommy!" I got a block away, and she's still standing there *screaming*, she's like this little kid in the distance. And I had to go back. In order to get her off the street I had to trick her, so I bought the ice cream, and when I took it home I told her she couldn't have it because she was bad, and I only bought the ice cream to get her off the street. It wasn't a good parenting technique, I mean it broke every rule of parenting, but it felt like life or death to me.

Having people see her difficulties with Lisa were a further shame for Esther:

> It was so humiliating. I couldn't *handle* my three-year-old you know, and the way people *looked* at me, oh, it was horrible! That was a very hard thing about having children, I didn't find that people were that nice to me about it. I mean here and there were people who were exceptionally nice, like there was one

Jehovah's Witness babysitter who used to help me out all the time. I ran into her recently, you know, she's just a beautiful woman, very spiritual, but I found a lot of people to act in a way that showed that they were sort of judging and horrified. When Lisa was a baby I had a housekeeper. I don't know why, but a neighbour approached the housekeeper and said, "I thank god that I'm not like that. But if I was like that I wouldn't have children." And the housekeeper repeated this to me, and I was devastated. I felt that people were looking at me and thinking, "Why did she reproduce [laugh]?" It was *so* horrible. I'm a very sensitive person, and I was sensing that some people were thinking, "That poor baby, that poor baby with that mother."

Esther's second child, Hannah, was born when Lisa was four and a half. The pregnancy was harder, the baby had pressed on a nerve so that she had trouble walking, but the birth was much better. By then, Esther was a little more knowledgeable about childbirth, and she also had an obstetrician she trusted. She decided that she wanted to have the baby vaginally:

He managed my labour to minimize the pushing. I mean, I was in labour for a long time and towards the very end, he gave me an epidural so I didn't push the baby out, the baby kind of slid out. It didn't feel so easy as that [laugh]! And that made my relationship with Hannah get off to a better start because I wasn't physically … you know — a Caesarean takes months to recover from, and vaginal delivery is twenty-four hours and you feel okay, and that made it a lot easier for me, much more fulfilling and exciting.

Esther found that mothering Hannah was much easier than it had been with Lisa, because Hannah was such a compliant, even-tempered baby. Hannah's birth also heralded a happier period in her marriage. Both she and Simon were so delighted to have two young daughters. This relative contentment, however, was short-lived. Before long, Simon once again began pressuring Esther to go back to work. Once again Esther did as he wanted:

A lot of the bad patterns started over again. He would call me a nasty bitch and a stupid fucking whore, and it was — well, [sigh] I felt totally trapped. Because he would say that if I left him, he would get the children because of my handicap, and I believed him. And I don't mean to paint a portrait of victimization but that's what it was like. And in a *way*, the most horrible thing about the stroke was that it opened me up to being trapped in an abusive relationship. I mean there were problems in my family in my childhood that certainly predisposed me as well, but had it not been for the stroke, I would have just not married him in the first place.

At the same time, Esther said that she is not sorry she married him, because not doing so would have meant "missing out on my wonderful children. So I'm not sorry; it was worth every moment of unhappiness."

She put up with the abusive relationship until her youngest was six and a half years old. By that time, the children were old enough that she felt she could manage them on her own. Esther had also become stronger within herself, so that Simon's threats of taking the children from her no longer scared her. She began to realize that she did not need "to be stuck with this man being abusive to me and feel that I had missed out on a chance for a loving relationship."

There is much in what Esther says about her marriage that is common among women struggling to leave abusive relationships. Abusive people, whether male or female, are often very good at honing in on someone else's weak spots and then blowing those weaknesses out of proportion, making the victim feel like she is to blame. Someone such as Esther, who was severely traumatized by the perceived losses that her stroke represented, such as her beliefs that she could no longer be independent and that she was no longer physically attractive, was especially vulnerable to abuse. Before she could leave Simon, she had to rebuild a sense of self-esteem — an uphill battle while being subject to ongoing emotional abuse.

When Esther left, after twelve years of marriage, Simon pleaded with her to give him another chance. He promised he would go to counselling and that he would change, but Esther said that, "by then, my heart had turned to stone, I couldn't deal with that." Leaving was very scary:

I felt like I was jumping off a cliff. And the first weeks were really hard. I mean, I had never had anything to do with finances, you know, taking care of the money stuff. The physical stuff, keeping the household going, was hard to adjust to. And my guilt about my children, fear of long-lasting trauma [for them] because of the divorce.

Moreover, she worried about her ability to care for her children on her own, given her physical impairments. Thus, she waited until the children were old enough to do things somewhat independently.

She and Simon ended up sharing custody of the children, an arrangement that Esther was happy with because it meant that the children would still live with her on a part-time basis. She also did not want them to be cut off from their father. Despite Simon's abuse of Esther, she thought he was an excellent father. Perhaps for this reason, the children did not understand why the divorce happened. From their uncritical perspective as children, they thought their father was wonderful. As Esther said:

I didn't tell my children why I was leaving their father behind, so they've absorbed this idea that I was crazy. He was not overt enough [with the psychological abuse], or bad enough, that they could see it. And maybe they just didn't want to see it. Because he happens to be an exceptionally good father, and so there was no reason why they *should* have seen the kind of husband that he was. And there was nothing served by them ever seeing it. So I had to be in the position of having them blame me for my decision.

As time went on, the children got used to moving back and forth between parents and stopped being angry at Esther. Life became easier, albeit full of the ups and downs that are inevitable for any mother of young children. At the time of the interview, Lisa was fifteen, and Esther said:

One thing that's interesting about Lisa's attitude about my stroke is she's not sympathetic. I mean, if I ask her to do something she'll come through, but she won't acknowledge that life is harder for me. My mother was trying to talk to her and say,

"You know, you have to give your mother a lot of credit for working after a stroke as well as she does." Lisa said, "Well, quadriplegics work." She doesn't see it, or she doesn't want to see it, I don't know what it is. She's a very perceptive person, but I think she's not that comfortable with the idea that I'm different, and so she doesn't want to see that my life is harder.

Esther's social circle was dramatically reduced after she left her husband. Although she had always kept in close touch with a group of women with whom she went to university, they lived all over the country so the relationships were long-distance. On a day-to-day basis, Esther found that the friends she and Simon had made, who were observant Jews, dropped her: "I didn't want to tell my story to a lot of people because of the kids, so no one knew quite why I left. Some people condemned me and rejected me and I felt like an outsider in the synagogue and I eventually dropped out. So I lost a community of friends."

Esther did manage to make new friends, but it was difficult because she is not by nature an outgoing person. After living on her own for a few years, she met a man she liked a lot and she invited him to move in with her. The relationship did not last long, though, and she ended up asking him to move out. She said:

> Part of the reason I think I chose this man who was really not right for me was because he was helping me with the housework. He would be around a lot and help take care of the house — somebody was helping me. But it turned out that he had an obsessive-compulsive disorder. When we met we had this bond because we'd both been through this thing with disability, trauma and hardship. After a time I found out that he kind of used his disability to retreat from the world and I didn't. I couldn't. I lost a lot of respect for him, because he was very hard to live with. He wanted all my attention when I walked through the door and I felt like I had a third child. I didn't want a forty-seven-year-old baby!

After he moved out, Esther was "just so happy to be left alone." Further, she no longer yearned for someone to help her.

> I hope to find love again someday, and I like men and I'm looking for companionship. But I know I'm just so far from feeling

that I won't survive without it. Actually, my mother helps me out. She's a very vigorous eighty-year-old woman who works out with a personal trainer and still drives, so she'll come once a week and pick up the kids from school and come and help out. I only have my children four nights a week at most, the rest of my time I have to myself. I spend a lot of that time just exhausted, I can't do as many fun things as I would like.

Esther stayed in her job as a librarian, partly because it paid well, and partly because she wasn't trained to do anything else. She became comfortable with her work, even though she did not find it completely fulfilling. Yet, by the time of the interview, at age forty-three, she was beginning to think seriously about what she could do to create a second career for herself:

I think I would have been a lot more successful in some career if I hadn't had the stroke. I think I would have had more strength to find something that was more fulfilling. I have a perfectly decent job, but I have a job that someone three years out of school could do. And it's a combination of the stroke and having had children. A lot of people are willing to sacrifice their children for their career and that was never an option for me. But had I not been physically limited, maybe I would have had more success with a change of professions. I feel bad about that, some days I feel very bad. Other days I feel like, you know, the acceptance and the spiritual growth make up for what I missed out on. I can be relatively philosophical but yeah, I haven't had the career that I might have had.

Nevertheless, Esther realizes that it's far from too late to change direction:

I've gained a lot of self-confidence since I left my husband. I was much different when I was married. More of a shadowy presence. Now from being on my own and kind of surviving, I'm starting to think about different things I'd like to do. And in a way, my experiences have given me a certain confidence that if I can survive a stroke and work and raise two children and then go and get a divorce and survive that, I can do anything!

Even if her life did not turn out as she might have envisioned before her stroke, Esther was, at the time of the interview, appreciative of all that she had. She suspected that if she had never had the stroke, she would have been a much shallower person. Instead, she said:

> It's made me much more compassionate. I was always smart and attractive and found it relatively easy living my life, and it certainly did make me a deeper person to have something absolutely terrible happen. It's definitely made me more spiritual, I needed more of a connection with God than I think I would have gotten if I hadn't had the stroke. So for the most part, it has changed me for the better.

*

After her stroke, it became Esther's task to use her intelligence to work at reimagining herself as a worthwhile person, not in spite of but *because of* her stroke. It's a struggle we all must engage in as we adapt to major changes and challenges in our lives. That Esther managed to do this was clear when I interviewed her. She had come to terms with the consequences of her stroke, and was in the process of creating a better, happier future for herself.

A few years after our interview, Esther met and married a loving, compassionate man. She remains happily married. There are echoes of Lauren Mayes's story here: both Esther and Lauren needed to develop a strong sense of self as competent women and needed to feel comfortable within themselves before they could establish a loving relationship with someone else.

Esther continues to share custody of her youngest daughter with her ex-husband. Her oldest daughter, meanwhile, has moved out to go to college, but in 2005, she became gravely ill. She had sudden liver failure and had to have a transplant. Esther found it exceedingly difficult to watch her nineteen-year-old daughter experience a trauma of similar magnitude to what she herself had experienced at a young age, but she also felt that her own journey through catastrophic illness gave her insight into what Lisa was going through, and perhaps helped her to be a more empathetic mother. Fortunately, her daughter has recovered. Another change in Esther's life is that she has quit her job and, after some rest time, plans to go into business for herself. She has been having health problems in recent years and finds that she no longer has the energy to work a nine-to-five job, five days a week. She is delighted to not have to go to work every day.

Chris Madsen

An Unusual Right-Handed Person: Disability and Identity

Chris Madsen had a hemorrhagic stroke due to an AVM rupture in 1990, at age twenty-five. In 1998, she published an abbreviated version of her story online. We struck up an e-mail correspondence, sharing our experiences with each other, trading stories about difficulties with everyday activities, and we learned that we had many things in common. For instance, we had both been affected with right-sided paralysis, we had both recovered to the point that others could not easily recognize our impairments, and we were both lesbians. I wasn't able to meet Chris in person until September 2002, when I travelled to her home in Springfield, Missouri. Chris is of Scandinavian heritage and was thirty-seven at the time of our interview.

Once she told me her story in-depth, I could see that an important theme in Chris's post-stroke life has been disability and identity. Much like I myself did, she spent the first few years after her stroke denying that she had permanent impairments that required her to reorganize how she did things. This denial was relatively easily accomplished, given that her impairments were mostly invisible to others. She did not want to be seen as different. Over the years, though, she has come to terms with her impairments and in so doing, she has become more comfortable identifying as disabled. Also significant in her story are the roles of support, career and rehabilitation. The following is based on her own writing, our correspondence and her interview with me.

*

Chris Madsen grew up in a small town in the American Northwest. The youngest of six children, she was the baby of the family. When she was nine years old her mother left for a relationship with another man, leaving Chris and her siblings with their father. Chris maintained a relationship with her mother, but emotionally she remained closer to her father. Financially, the family had ups and downs. For a while, her father had a well-paying job but then his employer went bankrupt. By the time Chris was old enough to go to college, he was struggling with his own business and wasn't able to pay for her education. She managed, nevertheless, to go to college by getting a series of grants and loans; she majored in English.

As she was finishing her last year of college, in Corvallis, Oregon, she did an internship at a TV station. Chris was fascinated by the whole process and wanted to learn more. So, she spent her last year at college learning all she could about videography, and when she graduated, she was offered a summer job as a photographer/videographer, making promotional videos for a large manufacturing firm. She eagerly accepted, and the job turned into something full-time and permanent.

Chris approached her job with determination and energy. A self-declared "type A personality," she "wanted to rule the world" and was doing her best to "rush up the ladder of success." Consequently, by age twenty-five she says, "I had ulcers. I was stressed out. I was working too much."

Part of her stress was also related to her recent decision to tell her parents that she was gay. For the preceding three years she had been in a relationship with Bev, a woman she had met at college, and they were living together. Chris was on good terms with her parents, but up to this point, she had not felt able to come out to them. A few, but not all, of her siblings knew. Bev, however, was very interested in being open about their relationship, and she pressured Chris to tell them. So, with trepidation, Chris sat down and wrote a coming-out letter to her parents. Her father took the news well. In fact:

> He called and said, "I wouldn't care if you walked hand in hand with a baboon." And that was nice, but I just don't think he ever really quite got it. But he seems fine, and then my mom, she freaked, she was like: "Oh my gosh, I've lost my baby, blah, blah, blah."

One of Chris's sisters intervened. Family friends had just suffered the death of their son, so Chris's sister pointed out that Chris was not dead, she was gay. Mrs. Madsen was not "losing" Chris. Chris thinks that it helped a lot to have it put like that, and her mother began to become more accepting. "The next thing I know," Chris said, "she's inviting Bev and me for breakfast." Two months later, in June 1990, Chris actually did almost die. In light of what happened, the matter of Chris's sexuality paled in comparison.

The morning Chris's AVM ruptured, causing a hemorrhagic stroke, she was out directing a live camera shoot. She wrote of that day:

> As I was directing the cameramen, my right arm began to go numb from my fingertips to my shoulder. I assumed it was a pinched nerve or something. But soon I knew something was really wrong when my right leg went out from under me. I called for help and this lady came to my assistance. At that moment I was mumbling and anxious. She thought I was having a nervous breakdown. The little town I worked in didn't have a hospital so the EMTs took me to the nearby town where doctors questioned my boss, my partner, my dad and tried questioning me to see what could have caused my condition (i.e., is she on drugs? could she be pregnant?) I just lay there not able to speak. I heard all the conversations and I just wanted to scream out things but I couldn't. No words could come.

They eventually did a CT scan and found the moderate bleed on the left side of my brain from the AVM. All I remember is the doctors putting my results on my stomach and wheeling me out to the ambulance as fast as they could because I had to be transferred to a neighbouring city. There I underwent emergency brain surgery.

In retrospect, Chris is grateful that her AVM ruptured while she was at work, because that meant there were other people around to ensure that she got help. She is frightened to think of what might have happened had she been alone. She is also glad that it happened after she had started a full-time job, because she had medical insurance through her employer. Insurance covered all of her hospitalization and rehabilitation expenses.

By seven that evening, Chris was recovering from her surgery. She spent the next week in hospital, feeling very uncomfortable. Her neck was very sore and every time she moved, it would crack and her monitors would start to beep. She got little sleep, even though she was being given lots of drugs. She was also visited several times by a physical therapist who would poke her to see what kind of movement she was capable of. Her doctors were not hopeful about the prospects for her recovery. They told her parents that, because the AVM had been near her speech centre, she might not regain the ability to talk coherently. They were similarly unhopeful about Chris being able to regain enough movement to walk without assistance.

She was transferred to a rehabilitation hospital, where she stayed for another month, relearning how to walk, talk and generally use her right side. Bev was constantly with her, and she had plenty of other visitors while she was in both the general and the rehabilitation hospital: family members (two of her sisters even stayed in her room for a few nights, sleeping on uncomfortable chairs), friends from work, her boss and her best friend from grade school came to see her:

When something like this happens to you, you don't even realize how many people know you, care about you or even have any interest whatsoever. I mean, after it happened, there were letters sent out to everybody updating them on how I was, people were bringing food for the family and the whole thing. There were lists of people, and I'm looking at this list, going, I hardly know her, you know. It was pretty cool. It was pretty awesome.

One of Chris's friends from work went so far as to bring in a video camera to record scenes from her stay at the rehabilitation centre. The video provides an interesting visual documentation of Chris's progress while in the hospital, and the sorts of things that she did there. In the beginning, her face and head were quite swollen and she could hardly do anything for herself. She did better once the swelling went away. Towards the end of her month-long stay she was walking unaided and was able to do things such as help wheel other patients to dinner.

Regaining physical movement was relatively easy for Chris. She thinks that this was because she was in excellent physical shape beforehand. Much more difficult for Chris to deal with was the "*terrible* aphasia" she had. Her ability to express herself verbally had been severely damaged, so that she "was really having a hard time thinking of words." She remembers speech therapy being quite difficult and she used to dread it because she felt so inadequate when she couldn't do what she thought should have been simple things. She was asked to describe objects and their use, such as a shoe, and was timed to see how long she took. Mostly, though, she had to work at talking coherently and intelligibly. For example, she would mix up sounds and letters. About this, she says:

> I had a couple of embarrassing moments — like, where did these words come from? Not like it's Tourette's or anything, but just mixing letters up. I was around a nurse and I said, "got my foot stuck" and somehow I got the "f" from "foot" to "stuck." It was bad! [laughter] We won't go there. But it was bad. Bev and I had a few laughs over that one!

She was not good at using words in their appropriate context, or she would insert words into her speech that were somewhat out of context. To some extent, she still has a problem with this. She explains:

It's like I've got these words up on the shelf. And out of the blue, all of a sudden, I'll insert a word into a sentence that makes no sense. I might be saying, you know, "the cow" and then finish what I was saying. Because the word was just there. It was just in the buffer, you know.

Chris was fortunate to have her friends and family around her to offer support, talk to her about what was going on and advocate for her with medical staff. Her difficulties with communication meant that she wasn't easily able to ask questions about what was going on around her or what would happen to her. At the best of times, when one is a patient in the hospital, staff often seem to have little time to answer one's questions. When the patient has aphasia, though, there is a very high likelihood that staff will not engage with attempts at communication. When one has aphasia, coupled with paralysis on one side of the face so that the very mechanics of forming words requires great effort, communication takes time and the listener needs to have patience. In Chris's case, she had to work hard at making herself understood, and it took time for that to happen. Her friends and family were willing to take the time necessary to listen to her. Chris, moreover, was fortunate that she had no real complaints about her hospital experiences. If she had, her difficulties with expressing her thoughts would have prevented her from being listened to by medical staff who were too busy to sit with her as she attempted to say what was on her mind.

The rehabilitation hospital was a well-organized centre with a variety of amenities to help patients recover. Such hospitals are relatively uncommon around the world — they tend to be newer and well-funded facilities, planned with a great deal of thought given to what is required to authentically simulate a non-hospital environment. Certainly, no one that I have ever talked to or interviewed about post-stroke experiences has mentioned having access to all of the features that were available to Chris. Many rehabilitation hospitals will have a heated pool, as it has long been understood that warm water provides an ideal environment in which to exercise stiff or atrophied muscles. But Chris also had access to a kitchen where she was expected to practise preparing meals, a mock store and areas set up as though they were street intersections. Chris was also periodically given tests to see how she was doing cognitively. She found these tests, which required her to do tasks such as sort objects and put them in order, or work with a chequebook, to be quite difficult. At the same time, she felt somewhat infantilized that at twenty-five years old, she was required to show others that she could do things that she had been doing for her whole life.

Altogether, the various types of therapy she got at the hospital made her very aware of how much she had lost as a result of the stroke. Yet, she says:

> What's weird is I never really had a black-and-white feeling about it. I didn't think, "Wow, I was in the hospital, boy, I'm going to have this rough road down the street, down the way, that I'm not going to be able to go to work like I used to, and do this and do this." I never expected that. I sort of expected that the next day would be all okay and I'd go back to work and life would be the same. I mean, call me naïve, but I had no clue for what seemed like some time, so it wasn't 'til I was there for a while and it occurred to me, "Oh yeah, this is a little hill here I have to get over."
>
> You know, my dad is such that he's a very positive guy and he'd say, "Oh, you can lick this, and if anybody can do this, you can do it." He wouldn't let me get into feeling poor me, poor me. And I'm the youngest of six kids, and they're all there and very helpful. I mean, you don't have time to be down when you've got all this support.

Nevertheless, some of the staff at the hospital were not supportive of Chris. There was one particular nurse who was a Christian fundamentalist, and she would say very disturbing things to Chris. Chris had shown her pictures from a recent vacation she had taken with Bev, and the nurse commented: "So how could a pretty girl like you be gay?" This nurse also suggested to her that she might have had the stroke because she was being punished for being gay. Then, the nurse would take Chris on walks around the grounds and lecture her:

She was very adamant about it. She'd be saying to me: "You know, you don't have to leave here the way you were when you came in," and stuff, and I was *so* freaked out. I mean I'm thinking: maybe I'm supposed to change, maybe this is a sign. I was just freaking out. I mean, the last week I told Bev not to even come over. You know, that's just *so* not right.

Chris had not, up to that point, felt that there was anything wrong with her sexuality. But in the hospital, still reeling from the trauma of her stroke, unable to care for herself, she was exceedingly vulnerable to the opinions of her caregivers. She wasn't in a position where she could ignore her nurse, much less engage in a debate with her. So, when she was alone, she could not help but wonder whether her nurse might be right. After she left the hospital, she was able to marvel at how emotionally abusive the nurse had been, but while she was there, she was too vulnerable to step back and see that the nurse had no right to pass judgement on her.

Chris and other patients were sometimes taken on outings in the "real world." A particularly memorable outing was when she was taken to a bowling alley for the first time. She recalls thinking that it would not be difficult for her to bowl, because she had been a good bowler before her stroke. The outing started out badly because the hospital bus was unavailable so everyone had to go by taxi. Chris bumped her head while getting in the taxi — an occurrence that led to her later spending time learning how to get in and out of a car. Then, when they got to the bowling alley:

I was thinking that everything was just going to be just fine. I'm like: "Oh, okay, I know what I'm doing." I didn't think about the fact that I had to put the ball on this right hand, so I was totally shocked. I couldn't bowl at all! You know, I couldn't believe it. So that opened my eyes big time. I'd get like a nineteen whole score, all together. And I'm used to about 139 or something. So it was tough.

The outings also exposed Chris to the way others were looking at her and the other patients. She felt self-conscious about her hair, because only half of her head had been shaved for surgery. She wondered what onlookers thought about her and the other patients. That too was an eye-opener for Chris, to experience being seen as different and possibly inferior.

After she was discharged from the hospital, she continued for a while with out-patient therapy. She found it particularly discouraging that, upon discharge, she could not go back to work right away or without assistance. She stayed off work for two months after leaving the hospital. Then, with the assistance of a job coach, she went back on a part-time basis for three months. In the state of Oregon, through the Office of Vocational Rehabilitation Services, job coaches are sometimes available to disabled people to help them with finding employment and performing employment-related duties. Typically, the job coach will closely monitor the client's work activities to see what is needed to help with job performance, will make recommendations about how tasks can best be completed and will work to facilitate a good working relationship between management and co-workers. As a state representative, the job coach can procure assistive technology and can arrange to have an employer modify job tasks. Chris, however, was not pleased with the idea of having a job coach and said:

> I thought I could go back to work full time and they were say-ing, "Uh, no, no, no." I didn't understand, I went through kind of an anger phase: "What? Why can't I come back to work?" Then they hired a — the state hired I guess — a job coach to follow me around for *way* too long. And that drove me crazy. She just followed me wherever I went. She didn't seem to help me but she kind of looked to see what I needed. I just remem-ber that was a really awkward time because I wanted to get back to normal, but I couldn't.

Here, we can see Chris feeling insecure about her abilities. The presence of the job coach was a clear reminder that she was not able-bodied as she had been before her stroke, and it was an affront to her dignity. She had yet to fully acknowledge that she was now a disabled woman. Chris was also feeling insecure because her employer had hired someone to fill in for her until she was able to come back to work full-time. But from her perspective, she saw it a bit differently:

He was this good-looking young guy who everybody loved because he was just real outgoing and I figured he was probably really, really good in his job as a videographer and stuff, and I was *very* intimidated by someone coming in and stealing the show and showing them that there's something better out there.

After three months of working part-time, Chris was thrilled to go back to work on a full-time basis. Especially for the first year after the stroke, she had significant impairments, but she was determined not to let them get in the way of what she wanted to do. Although naturally right-handed, she learned to do a lot of things with her left hand. She never gave up trying to use her right hand, though, and continues to think of herself as right-handed:

I utilize my left hand a ton with things that I used to do with my right. So I would say I use my left hand a *lot* more than I used to, so I'm kind of an unusual right-handed person because I use my left a lot. People are always saying, "Oh, you're left handed?" I'm like, "No, not really."

For about two years after her stroke, Chris noticed steady improvements in her balance and her ability to co-ordinate movements on her right side. After that, improvements came more slowly. She got to the point where others would not notice that she was having difficulty doing anything, even though, twelve years after her stroke, she continues to have significant right-sided weakness. Regardless of what others see or think, she herself knows that there are things she used to be able to do that she can no longer do. She is reminded on a daily basis of her limitations, in the course of performing activities as mundane as brushing her teeth, an activity for which she now must use her left hand. She is no longer eager to play softball — an activity she used to enjoy considerably. Now she finds it embarrassing because she can't throw a ball very well. Similarly, taking photographs — an activity that is an important part of her work — is not as simple to do as it once was, and she has adapted how she does this. She is also aware of a tendency to drag her right foot when she is tired, although she doesn't do this as much as she used to.

More disconcerting for Chris are the continued cognitive

difficulties she has. They are subtle, mostly not noticed by anyone else, but she is acutely aware of them. Her memory, she says, is terrible. She often has trouble expressing ideas, and she can become easily confused. If she is talking about something but becomes momentarily distracted by another thought, she has trouble remembering where she was going with the original thought. It's as though thoughts are "directional lines" and if she strays off the path, she won't be able to find her way back to where she was. Further, she explains, fatigue worsens the difficulties: "If I'm tired, I can't think for anything. I can't speak real well. So if I'm exhausted or something or have a lot of things on my mind, it's really hard for me to grab the words I need. Or if I'm stressed out."

In other areas of her life, Chris has continued to grow and find greater satisfaction. About a year after Chris's stroke, she broke up with Bev. The relationship — a first lesbian relationship for both women — had been "one of those college situations" and there had always been ups and downs. Chris had never been comfortable with what she saw as Bev's tendency to be confrontational about their sexuality. She strongly disagreed with Bev's belief that they should "come out to the world." She was more interested in being discreet — in part she did not want to upset anyone, but she also felt that her private life was no one's business but her own. Chris, therefore, had been very uncomfortable when she was in the rehabilitation hospital and Bev would talk to staff about Chris being her spouse. "So," Chris said, "we struggled in those areas."

The relationship finally ended after Bev made plans to go away to study for her Master of Arts degree. In retrospect, Chris says that "it was an excellent first relationship in many ways," but "also it was not good in some because I was trying to figure out who I was, and I felt like at many times that she had too much control." She believes it was "for the best" that they did not stay together.

As time went on, Chris developed more confidence in herself and became clearer about what she was looking for in a partner. At the time of her interview, she had been living very happily with Michelle for more than two years.

Chris's work situation, meanwhile, steadily improved after she went back full-time, almost six months after her stroke. She was then twenty-six, and was good at what she did. In fact, she was so good at making videos that when her boss decided to take a job in a midwestern city, he invited Chris to move with him so that she could continue to work for him as a videographer. The position didn't actually exist, but he wanted to create it for Chris. At first, Chris was not sure that she wanted to move to a different part of the country. She was happy in her small town, surrounded by her family. Her boss talked her into it, though, so in 1996 she moved to Springfield, Missouri, to begin a new life.

Unlike the case at her former workplace, the new job involves occasional travel both inside and outside North America. About this, Chris says:

> In the first couple years I got to go to four European branches and I've been to the Thailand branch, and we have branches all around the United States, so I've been able to go to several of those from the West Coast to the East Coast. I mean, I've been very fortunate, even though it's been a ton of work. I go by myself, I carry all the stuff. It's really hard work and it's not glamorous whatsoever. It sounds better than it is. But it's been a great experience.
>
> I went to Europe for three weeks — first time out of the country, except for British Columbia. I went by myself, with all my equipment to four countries, with four types of money, four languages, and I thought if I can do this, I can do anything. Then when I went to Thailand, same thing. It was *tough*! And so it's kind of a neat little thing, I felt pretty strong about that. Because I — it's scary, I mean, I might be an extrovert but, you know, I prefer to have the comfort of home too. But it was a lot of fun.

At the same time, Chris generally finds it somewhat unsettling to be required to work with new people all the time. She says:

> I've always found that every time I'm in a new situation, dealing with an administrator or one of the branch directors or something, I always wonder: "Can they tell?" Because I slur words sometimes or I can't think of words. I feel a little bit off

sometimes. And I wonder: "What is their perception? Do they think I don't have everything upstairs? Am I completely there?" So, I do my best to cover up any of the issues with that, but I definitely feel that way.

She remains very conscious of the fact that she does things differently than she used to. As she says, "I mean, every single day I do notice that there's a difference." She is surprised, then, when others say they don't notice anything unusual about how she does things. At the same time, though, she is happy not to be the focus of attention. She can become quite uncomfortable when others, upon learning of her stroke and impairments, suggest that there is something special about what she has done. She tells the following story to illustrate:

We have some lesbian neighbours across the street and we had dinner with them one night, and we were talking about our families. "Oh how many kids are in your family?" "Oh this many, but my brother died." "Oh yeah, how?" "Aneurysm." You know, I *hate* that. You know, I'm having this nice dinner and I'm suddenly reminded that I made it through. And I sort of feel guilty in some ways even though I'm happy I didn't die, obviously.

Now some people say, "Well you really had a lot of determination and look at how well you've done or whatever." And I'm thinking, "Well, to be honest, I don't think I've really kicked butt on it or anything to get through this. I think I really went through it at a normal pace." I think, "Okay, I had this happen, I think I need to go through it." And you know, it's hard to explain that to others so they'll understand.

This is not to say that Chris is nonchalant about what happened to her. She recognizes that "it *is* a big deal." Chris does not minimize her stroke, her recovery process or the impact that this has had on her life. The scar that is hidden under the hair on her head from the brain surgery — which she thinks is "cool" — serves as a visceral reminder of what happened. Yet, when she considers the impact that the stroke had on her life, she considers how her approach to life has changed. She says:

I'm pretty sure I would be a different person. 'Cause I mean, I was pretty much a Type A personality, go, go go, who knows where! I couldn't allow myself to relax. Now, I enjoy life a little bit more, I appreciate people more, I appreciate my family more. I really think it's made me stronger and a stronger spiritual person. I'm much more thankful for what I have and very thankful to be where I am and have everything that's in my life.

A few years into her new job, Chris decided that she wanted to get her master's degree in media communications. She enrolled in the program but was worried about her ability to cope with all the writing that would be required. She knew, for example, that if she had to write a test she would not be able to write legibly. So she went to the Academic Resources Centre for help, and got permission to type her tests. It was an accommodation that Chris needed, but she was also acutely aware that some of her professors were not happy with being asked to adjust their expectations. "Some of the professors just didn't get it," she said. "It was kind of a big deal for some of them, like a real inconvenience. It really made me feel uncomfortable but it was one of those things where it would have been even worse if I had to handwrite these essay questions."

In this manner, Chris ended up getting her degree. Along the way, she became acquainted with disability politics. She was first invited by someone at the Academic Resources Centre to join the university's accessibility committee. It sounded intriguing to Chris, so she joined. Then she found that the issues resonated with her so much that she stayed involved. For a while, she even chaired the committee, but she found that getting anything done was a matter of politics, and it was frustrating to have no power. She happily passed on the chair to a faculty member, therefore, who would have a voice within the university hierarchy and might have been better able to get things done.

Even though Chris became disabled when she had her stroke, it took a while before it really sunk in for her that her life would never be the same as it was before she had the stroke. In fact, when she was first released from the rehabilitation hospital, she recalls: "I got this little thing from the hospital when the vocational rehab people hired that job coach. And it did say something like 'you're disabled.' And I said, 'Huh, how long does that last? I mean, won't I get better?'"

Over time, though, as she worked at recovery, she learned to adapt and integrate into her life new ways of being. The process has allowed her to move towards an empathetic appreciation for the situation of other disabled people. She feels that she has an understanding of the issues and that she has something in common with people who are more disabled than she is. She has, in fact, become quite passionate about the need to improve disabled access at her university:

> I do feel for people who are in a wheelchair. And our campus is so backwards, there isn't a lot of accessibility and there's just none in some areas. We have some really old buildings so it's hard to do anything with them. They give you this wheelchair lift but then there's no way to get in this one door and things like that. You know, if any of these administrators were in a wheelchair, they would *never* allow this to be. So that's why I've been a little more adamant. And they didn't see that there was a problem with having only two accessible parking spots! They said they took up a lot of room, and there were a lot of times during they day when they weren't being used.

Chris feels fortunate in her life — fortunate to have survived her AVM rupture, fortunate to have friends along with a large and loving family to help her recover, fortunate to have a job she loves and fortunate to have a loving partner with whom she can envision sharing the rest of her life. It's not that her impairments are of no consequence to her, it's that she does not define herself by what she cannot do. As she once wrote:

> I have no bitterness for having this happen to me. It just opened my eyes to a lot. It really reminded me of the little things we often take for granted. It helped me slow down, become more real and down to earth. My life may have been changed considerably back in 1990, but I have to say, it has changed for the better in many ways.

*

Chris remains close to her family and continues to visit them whenever she can. Yet it seems significant that it was only after her cross-country move placed her in a new environment that she really began to acknowledge how she had been changed by the stroke. Sometimes it can be hard to reinvent ourselves when surrounded by people we have known all our lives. Moving away, at first knowing no one but her boss, Chris could imagine herself anew, as Lauren Mayes did when she travelled to Belize. In Springfield, Chris was able to "come out" as a disabled woman, even if that coming out was mostly to herself. No longer does she dream of returning to her pre-stroke life and body. Instead, she has become comfortable with who she is — and that includes recognizing that her impairments are an important part of her.

Since our interview in 2002, Chris has continued to enjoy her work as a videographer and she remains involved in advocating for disability rights. Her relationship with Michelle has grown deeper and stronger over the years, and in 2006 she and Michelle became mothers. Chris is so proud of her new daughter that she has created a Web page, complete with video, photos and text, to document and celebrate her birth and life.

Katherine Price

Adjusting to a New Future:
Independence and Dependence

Katherine Price was twenty-eight years old when she had a hemorrhagic stroke due to a ruptured aneurysm in 2000. In the spring of 2005, I visited her at her home in the small town of Pomona, New York, in the northeastern United States, where she lives with her parents. When I arrived, she introduced me to her mother and father and we went into the kitchen to talk alone, while drinking coffee and munching on the muffins that she had laid out. Katherine, who is Italian-American, was thirty-three at the time of the interview.

Unlike most of the other women in this book, Katherine is still in the process of adjusting to the consequences of her stroke. Before her stroke, she was an independent, upwardly mobile career woman. Post-stroke, she has become dependent on her parents because she is unable to work. Going from a sense of independence to a sense of dependence can be an enormous challenge to one's sense of self, and it's this that Katherine continues to negotiate. Issues around career and work, loss and depression, faith, support and financial resources are also illuminated by Katherine's story.

*

Katherine Price was a career-oriented young woman who was enjoying life. She had a master's degree in art therapy, and worked with children who had serious medical problems. She advocated on their behalf with doctors and felt strongly that it was important for medical personnel to take the children's emotional well-being into account as they treated their physical conditions. She also taught art therapy to university students. She loved working with children, and she loved teaching. She had aspirations of becoming chairperson of the art therapy program at the university.

Katherine had been living on her own since she was eighteen. Before she left home, she'd worked hard each summer to save, anticipating the day when she would be able to afford her own apartment. She was a very self-sufficient young woman, and even though her parents wanted to help her with things, she cherished her independence. She had put herself through university with student loans and was in the process of paying them back.

Katherine spent her free time travelling and pursuing her interest in photography, both of which she loved to do. Her social life was good, and she enjoyed dating, but she had never really had a serious, long-term relationship with a man. The longest romantic relationship she had ever been in had lasted for nine months. She was more interested in having good friends than in settling down with someone. She was entirely too focused on her career and her independence to worry about serious romance.

In early 2000 Katherine started going to Tai Chi classes. She found the practice very helpful for dealing with the stress that was an inevitable part of her work. That September, she started a new class at a nearby hospital, but halfway through the very first class, she collapsed. She vaguely recalls coming to again, but her memories of what happened after that are not at all clear.

After Katherine collapsed, she was immediately taken to the emergency room. Once there, she remembers the emergency personnel repeatedly asking her if she was pregnant, and asking her other questions as they tried to determine what had happened. She also remembers that by this time she was vomiting a lot, but she does not recall having a headache. Soon enough, though, she was sent for a CT scan and her ruptured aneurysm was discovered. Katherine was only semi-conscious through all of this. Yet when her hemorrhagic stroke was discovered, she was able to request a transfer to the hospital where she worked. Partly she wanted to go there because she knew people at that hospital, but also it was a large and well-equipped hospital so she knew she would get good care.

She was transferred by ambulance, and the next day, she had surgery to repair her ruptured aneurysm. She has little memory of being prepared for the surgery or recovering from it, but she has been told that she did not do well after the surgery, which likely means that she was not responding as expected in terms of vital signs and return to consciousness. That evening she became delirious. She was then put into an induced coma so that her brain could be protected while healing from the surgery. Nevertheless, Katherine developed hydrocephalus (brain swelling, due to fluid build-up), and she had to have a second operation to insert a shunt so that fluid could be drained away from her brain. She was also put on a ventilator and given a tracheotomy and a feeding tube. About two weeks after her hemorrhagic stroke, she had a vasospasm (narrowing of the arteries) which caused an ischemic stroke (a complication that sometimes occurs after hemorrhagic stroke). With all of these problems, Katherine was in the intensive care unit for two months. She remembers little about being in ICU. She has only snapshot-like memories of things happening, such as having blood taken or seeing someone she knew. She thinks she got very good treatment, though, because she had friends and colleagues who worked there, who were continually monitoring how she was doing. She said:

> From what I have been told, they even had prayers for me at the hospital church, they would come and sing when I was in the coma, give me hand massages and paint my nails. Too bad that I didn't respond to this attention! But, then again, I have heard that I didn't like anything on my body — pulling my trach, peg, gowns, etc. I didn't want it so I pulled things away. So I guess I was a pain in the butt.

When she was deemed stable, she was transferred to a rehabilitation hospital where she stayed for another two months. She was completely paralyzed on her right side, she was still on a feeding tube, and she had severe aphasia. Katherine couldn't understand what had happened to her, even though everyone tried to explain it to her. Although she didn't name the specific type of aphasia she had, it seems likely that she had what is known as global aphasia, which is the total, or near total, loss of the ability to use language. People with global aphasia have great difficulty understanding what other people are saying, and they are unable to express themselves as well. Katherine recalled:

> They told me that I'd had an aneurysm and a stroke, but I couldn't connect the two. How could I have an aneurysm *and* a stroke at the same time? And I had no clue with the tracheotomy and they shaved all my hair and I remember — I just see little pictures, like when I was at physical therapy I'm in the wheelchair and I'm looking at a mirror, and I'm looking at me with no hair or anything and I couldn't realize that that was me. I couldn't, I *really* couldn't communicate whatsoever, but in my *mind*, I was saying, like what is their problem? What's happening? And then I would cry when I would ask what happened and they said it's the aneurysm and I said, "Does my mom know this, does my dad know this?" So I never really understood.

Katherine's strongest memory from her time at the rehab hospital was the poor treatment she received from the hospital aides. She said:

> I didn't like the aides. They didn't know anything about aphasia. They just pushed you around every so often, 'cause I couldn't get up, they'd wake you up, they would dress me up, they would get me ready — I couldn't do anything. But after a while, I found certain aides every so often that they could respond to me.

Katherine had physical, occupational and speech therapy there. Slowly she regained the use of her right side and began to walk again. She went from needing to use a wheelchair to being able to walk with a cane and a brace on her right leg and foot. She was told by her physical therapist when she left the rehab hospital that she should only use the brace when she was going to walk a long distance. She was also given a brace to wear on her foot at night, but she found it so uncomfortable to sleep with that when she got home she threw it away.

She had a lot of speech therapy at the rehab hospital to help her deal with her aphasia, and slowly she was able to make progress with her ability to express herself. In this regard, she was not unlike other stroke survivors who experience severe aphasia immediately following a stroke, but who manage over time to recover some or most of their ability to understand others and express themselves. While the physiology of what exactly happens is still not completely understood (so much of how the brain functions remains a mystery), it might be useful to think of the language functions in the brain as going into shock due to the trauma of stroke, but they are capable of recovering, or other parts of the brain take over to compensate for the loss of language abilities. For the person living with aphasia, as Katherine was and is, the experience is exceedingly unsettling. Aphasia does not compromise intelligence, it only compromises the ability to show evidence to others of intelligence. Thus, it is frustrating to know things, inside oneself, but be unable to express what one knows because one does not know how to access the appropriate words or language to use. Similarly, it is frustrating to listen to someone speak, or read what someone has written, and recognize the words used but be unable to figure out how those words are connected to mean something. The experience is an isolating one, and certainly affects one's sense of being able to negotiate the world as a self-sufficient individual.

Katherine also worked with a neuropsychologist who tested her cognitive abilities, but she found this very unhelpful. She would get very negative results from the tests that she was given, and she felt that she wasn't being given the help she needed to learn to express herself coherently. She felt as though she was being written off as a lost cause.

Occupational therapy was also difficult for Katherine because of the assumptions that the therapists were making about what she could do. In particular, she was encouraged to train for a low-paying job. She said:

> They wanted you to do vocational stuff and I was so annoyed and angry — because why did I work so hard and now have them tell me to work at McDonald's or A&P? Even the neuro-psychologist wasn't good. Um, they just assumed that this is the way my life was going to be, and like it happened to you when you were young and it's *sad* and that's it. They just wanted me to do vocational stuff. Funny things that I really didn't want to do.

Just as Lauren Mayes had been thirty years earlier, Katherine was advised to move in to a nursing home upon leaving the hospital. Rehabilitation professionals seemed to Katherine to assume that she was facing a lifetime of physical and cognitive impairment that would never improve. This is hardly a recipe for encouraging survivors to feel good about themselves. Rather, survivors such as Katherine are still getting the message that they are deluded if they think they are ever going to get any better. There is an amazing lack of sensitivity to the thoughts or feelings of survivors, and there is an amazing disregard of the now considerable evidence that shows survivors can, with concentrated effort, learn to minimize the disabling consequences of aphasia and can continue to regain physical function for years after a stroke. If nothing else, most of the stories in this book are evidence of that. Surrounded by negativity, however, many survivors are subtly encouraged to give up. Fortunately, Katherine did not give up.

After two months at the rehab hospital, dissatisfied with the therapy she was getting, Katherine discharged herself and went to live with her parents. She continued going to therapy as an outpatient. Her father, or sometimes her brother, would drive her there. She spent the next year going to physical therapy three times a week. At first, she was very optimistic about her prospects for making a complete recovery and regaining her pre-stroke abilities. It wasn't until after she had been out of the hospital for about six months that she began to understand the significance of what had happened to her and that she was not likely to ever recover all her abilities. "I thought that if I do all the exercises everything will be fine," she explained. "I was out for lunch, I guess. It took me forever just to say the word aneurysm, let alone stroke, let alone understand what the words mean."

Katherine's doctor, meanwhile, was an internist who was also skilled in acupuncture, so she was able to have many acupuncture treatments that were 80 percent covered by her insurance. These treatments, she said, were enormously helpful in allowing her to not only regain physical movement but also her ability to talk more or less fluently. Katherine was very fortunate to have a medical doctor who was trained in acupuncture techniques, as this is not a commonly used treatment for stroke rehabilitation. Acupuncture is considered a type of "complementary and alternative medicine," and there are few medical insurance plans that will cover the cost of treatment, despite evidence that acupuncture can be very helpful for treating a wide variety of medical concerns.

She stopped going to physical therapy after she was fitted with an AFO (an ankle foot orthosis, which helps stabilize and support the foot and ankle) and was able to walk without a cane. Katherine probably would have kept going, but once she was able to walk without the cane, her therapist felt that she no longer needed to go, and her insurance would no longer cover the sessions. For her part, Katherine felt that there was still a lot of work that she had to do in order to improve her walking and her ability to use her right side. Undaunted, she took out a membership in a gym and started going three times a week to practise her exercises. She spent about an hour and a half there each time.

Dealing with her aphasia was especially hard for Katherine. She went to speech therapy at the rehab hospital as an outpatient, but was very dissatisfied. She was put in a group with about fifteen people, and the therapy focused on cognitive skills. Katherine was more interested in developing her ability to express herself, and she felt that she wasn't able to do that in the group setting. About nine months after her stroke, Katherine was retested by the neuropsychologist. The test results were very discouraging, and Katherine even felt embarrassed to see a report that rated her cognitive skills at below average. She had trouble understanding why she had aphasia, or how it was possible that she could do so poorly on cognitive tests given that she was a well-educated woman who had previously held down a demanding job.

Katherine does not know the names of the cognitive tests she was given, but it is likely that she was given tests that rely heavily upon linguistic processing, as these are the most commonly used tests. The reliance on verbal stimuli and linguistic materials, however, means that such tests cannot easily distinguish between poor performance due to cognitive problems and poor performance due to aphasia. Given that aphasia is a language and communication disorder, it doesn't seem to make a lot of sense to test cognitive skills in people with aphasia by asking them to rely upon the ability to express oneself and understand language.

Katherine knew that the hospital she was going to had a very good reputation, but she felt it was undeserved. She stopped going to the group sessions and sought out a speech therapist of her own for individual sessions. This required her paying for the therapy on her own, rather than being able to have it covered by her insurance, but she believes it was worth the cost. She was, by then, receiving disability benefits from the insurance policy she had while employed, and she used that income to pay for the therapy. She was able to use her income to do this because she was living with her parents and not required to pay rent.

She did make progress when working on a one-to-one basis, and continued seeing a speech therapist for two years. Then, when she stopped seeing a therapist, she decided to start volunteering at a place for people with dementia and Alzheimer's disease. She would go there just to practise her communication skills, and did this for about a year. It was a wonderful place for her to rehearse ways of expressing herself, because the people with whom she was talking were non-judgemental. If she took longer than non-aphasic people to make herself understood, or if she made grammatical mistakes while talking, no one thought less of her. She could sit in that nonthreatening environment and communicate with other people who had communication difficulties themselves. The non-judgemental environment was important for building her confidence and sense of self-esteem. Elsewhere, she felt (and still feels) others were looking at her negatively on account of her language difficulties. She said: "You feel weird saying the wrong words or if you can't find what you are trying to say. Or intimidated. For me, I always feel intimidated, very easily."

During the months when Katherine was too aphasic to understand what had happened to her or what was going on, she was motivated to participate in various therapies because she thought she would return to life as it had been before her stroke. Once she understood that her impairments were more or less permanent, she felt angry. Yet she remained motivated to regain as much as possible. She wanted her independence back, and she was prepared to do all she could to get there.

Katherine found that one of the effects of the stroke was that she became easily exhausted. When she moved in with her parents upon leaving the hospital, therefore, she relished her ability to be able to take a nap for as long as she wanted. It was not unusual for her to go to her therapy session and then go home to sleep for four hours or more. She also decided that she would start doing things that she had wanted to do before the stroke but had never had time to do. When she came home, she said, "I really got into gardening and doing all these things that I wanted to do for fun. I would do cooking and tons in the garden." At the same time, she said, "I did it, but it was more like a task. Like, chalk [check] it off I did *that*, I did *that*, I did *that*." Although she could take satisfaction from accomplishing tasks, she was simultaneously focused on trying to push herself to do more, so it was difficult to really enjoy what she was doing.

It was not easy for Katherine to move in with her parents, since she had left home ten years before. Although she was extremely grateful to them for all the help they were giving her, she was used to living independently, and especially during the first few months at home, she couldn't really understand why she had to stay with them. As well, her difficulties with expressing herself meant that there were frequent misunderstandings between her and her parents. Katherine would think she was saying something but they would not respond as she expected.

Her communication difficulties, which were both frustrating and depressing, led Katherine to start seeing a psychologist. Her insurance paid for her to see the psychologist weekly for a month and a half, and then Katherine had to pay for it herself. So, she went once every two weeks for a while, but because of the expense, eventually stopped going. She found the sessions with the psychologist helpful for learning how to come to terms with all that had happened to her. Stroke is, after all, a traumatic event. Frustration and depression are very common reactions, and psychotherapy can be quite helpful for stroke survivors as they struggle with these emotions. Psychotherapy, however, is rarely recommended by doctors (which is required for any kind of insurance to cover or contribute towards the costs). This means that few stroke survivors are likely to be aware of the potential benefits of psychotherapy, or if they are, they may not have the financial resources to pay for it. It remains the case that there is a stigma associated with mental illness (depression, of course, is a form of mental illness). Few people want to acknowledge that they need help dealing with emotions. Katherine was more willing to look for help, though, because in her career she had worked closely with psychologists and knew first-hand how they could help people.

As her aphasia became less severe and Katherine was able to both understand what was going on and was able to express herself with more clarity, she started to feel better about herself. She was also seeing continual improvement in her physical abilities. After two years, she had recovered enough control over her right side to start driving again. This did wonders for her sense of independence. She began to think about what kind of work she wanted to do, given her impairments. She couldn't go back to being an art therapist, because that job required the ability to think and act quickly, and generally be responsive to those with whom she worked. With aphasia, Katherine no longer had those abilities.

Just as Katherine seemed to be getting back on an even keel, about three years after her stroke, she developed a new problem:

> I was walking in the mall and my foot just stopped, I couldn't do anything. And then it was actually happening on my *left* too, up to my knee, and I would just stop and I couldn't do anything and then I'd get panicky and then I'd hold onto something. And then it sort of just disappeared. But then I went to [my volunteering] and I walked out to that *big* parking lot, and I was walking and then all of a sudden I got that paralyzing feeling and then there's nothing for me to hold on to. I tried to talk myself down, calm down, 'cause I didn't want to fall or collapse or anything.

Katherine went to her doctor about this new problem, and she was given a diagnosis of vertigo. At first, this seemed to make sense, as she became dizzy and easily unbalanced while walking in open spaces. For a while she would even become dizzy while standing in her own bedroom and would need to hold onto something. Eventually, she learned that she needed to find something to focus on, and that would help her with being able to walk without losing her balance. But it also became clear that vertigo was not her only problem, that there was something else going on with her leg muscles that was impairing her ability to walk. Almost a year after she first noticed this new problem, she saw a new doctor and was diagnosed with the neurological disorder dystonia (involuntary and sustained muscle contractions).

No one can tell Katherine why she has developed dystonia, or why it took so many years after her stroke to become a problem. All the doctors can tell her is that it is a common neurological disorder, but that is of little comfort to Katherine who finds that her ability to go where she wants has been seriously restricted. Thanks to the dystonia, she has stopped driving. She is going to physical therapy again, and she is also getting botox injections once every three months. Since she no longer has private insurance coverage, she is paying for these therapies herself, out of her disability benefit cheque that she receives from the government.

She knows that she is fortunate to have the money to do this, thanks to her parents' willingness to let her live at home rent-free. Both the physical therapy and the botox treatments are helping a great deal to control the disabling consequences of dystonia.

She also started seeing a psychologist again, because she became very depressed after developing dystonia. She wasn't able to afford to pay the psychologist on her own, and so she applied to a state-run program that assists brain-injury survivors, and she was given enough funding to cover weekly sessions for three months, and then bi-weekly sessions for another two months. About her need for psychological counselling, she said:

I had to stop *everything*. I was always crying all the time. And I would always be really pessimistic and then I'd talk about what I used to be, the whole thing, the old versus the new. It's like my body wasn't working with me, with the dystonia. I was trying again and it's just everything's falling apart, and it felt like I was going backwards.

The doctor put Katherine on antidepressant medication, which she finds helpful. While she continues to have times when she feels depressed, she no longer gets stuck in that set of feelings. She even feels optimistic about the future.

To some extent, when Katherine feels down she is able to find comfort in her religious beliefs. She was raised Catholic but before the stroke she mostly went to church only on the major holidays. Since the stroke, though, she has been going regularly:

I spend more time going to church. It makes me think. Not that I'm Miss Catholic but I try to understand some meaning. And faith, the whole thing with faith, that's a big thing for me ever since. Yeah. It's almost like I can get into a conversation, trying to figure out why this is happening and what's going on. I'm always thinking.

Her faith, she said, has given her the inner strength to keep pushing to recover as much as she can.

Katherine had a lot of friends before her stroke, and she was able to keep many of these friendships. Her friends have been very important to her throughout her recovery process. Yet she is also losing old friends as they move on with their lives, leaving Katherine behind. Katherine is mostly philosophical about this, seeing it as inevitable that her friendships change as circumstances change. She believes in synchronicity — that things happen when they should and that the right people will come into her life at the appropriate time. She does not simply wait for people to come into her life, though. Rather, she tries to put herself in social situations where she will meet people. She talks to people at the gym, for instance, and over the years she has joined a number of support groups hoping to meet others with whom she can establish friendships. Her experiences with groups, however, have not been very satisfying.

The first support group she joined was one for people who've had an aneurysm. She didn't go to that group for very long, though, as she didn't find it very supportive. She explained:

> First of all, people didn't actually *go*, maybe there was like two other people. It wasn't a real group. And if they went, they minimized what I went through and then I felt like I needed to show them what I went through. You know, someone had *five* aneurysms. Well, you had five aneurysms, but you're fine. I can't walk, I can't do this, and I just didn't know how to explain my problems.

Then, after she had been home for a while, her speech therapist suggested she go to a brain-injury support group. Although she found that she had more in common with the people who went there, the group met only once a month and she found it hard to feel connected to them. Also, there was little continuity in terms of who went each month. The first two times she went, there were young men there who had been injured in accidents, and the third time she went a lot of people were there, but they were all much older than Katherine. Because of her communication problems, she found it difficult to find space to tell her own story, and when she did get a chance to talk about herself, she couldn't figure out what to say. She does better, she says, talking to someone on a one-to-one basis.

The third support group was for stroke survivors, but this

group was made up exclusively of older survivors. She found that because they had had a stroke in old age, they had a very different attitude towards their strokes. They didn't seem to Katherine to be interested in talking about what they wanted to do with their lives. Rather, they seemed to have the attitude that, because they were already old, their lives were over and it was just a matter of waiting to die. Again, Katherine found that she couldn't identify with the other participants.

Eventually, she stopped going to support group meetings, but she doesn't regret the times she went. She thinks it's good to get out and meet people. At the time of the interview, she was going regularly to an exercise class for stroke survivors, which she enjoyed. Everyone there was much older than Katherine, but she felt comfortable doing exercises with them and chatting. The casual interaction was extremely important to Katherine, as she had precious few opportunities to meet and talk to other stroke survivors face to face.

She began to realize that she was more comfortable with the older people than with people her own age. They were patient with her, and she could relax without being concerned about whether she was walking properly, whether she might have a dizzy spell or whether she was making sense in what she was saying. Sometimes, someone else will tell her that they know a young man who's single that Katherine might enjoy meeting. But she never follows up on this, because she is too self-conscious about her impairments. With people her own age, unless they are themselves disabled, she feels nervous and afraid that she won't be accepted for who she is.

Once she went out to meet a young man her own age who had aphasia. Her speech therapist had introduced them. They both had a different agenda, though; he was looking for a romantic relationship, whereas Katherine was just looking for friendship. When he called her to ask her to go out for dinner and to a movie, Katherine felt overwhelmed. She told him that she wanted to get to know him better before she went out for dinner with him, and she suggested that they meet for coffee instead. He agreed, and Katherine felt they had an interesting conversation that could lead to continued friendship, but he apparently was uninterested in just a friendship. So, they didn't see each other again. Still, Katherine felt that she would like to meet others her own age who have impairments.

When Katherine discovered the StrokeNet Web site for young stroke survivors, she was delighted. The site, which maintains an active discussion board and chat room, has been a key factor in reducing her sense of isolation, and she checks it regularly to see what others are talking about. She occasionally posts her own thoughts on the discussion board, and she often sends welcome messages to newcomers. She knows from her own experience how important it is to feel supported by others. She has developed some e-mail friendships with others who are close to her own age and maintains private correspondence with them. She is thrilled to be able to interact, if only via e-mail, with others her own age who understand what she is going through: "Just to share people's stories to learn that you're not the only one. That's the biggest thing, and everyone is different."

Although Katherine's aphasia means that she can find it difficult to read, she reads as much as she can on the discussion board. Writing an e-mail message is a little easier for her than reading, but that too can be hard work, and she likes that she can take her time writing something without feeling pressure:

> I love being able to interact on the computer. And if I write it wrong, there is the famous "delete." But in reality a delete is hard when you are talking to people face to face or on the phone. The words have completely come out and how do you undo something? Miscommunication, to say the least!

Katherine also attends an annual conference for people with aphasia, which she always finds empowering because she can meet and interact with others who have aphasia and learn from their experiences. One year she was very excited at the workshop to meet someone in person whom she had first met on the Internet discussion board. Much as she likes being able to communicate with others via e-mail, she still yearns to talk to others in person.

Now that Katherine is on antidepressant medication, she is able to feel more positive about herself and make plans for the future. Her medication doesn't rob her of the ability to intensely feel emotional highs and lows, as can happen to people on antidepressants. Rather, it allows her to gain control of her thinking patterns:

> Before the medicine I tended to think about it over and over and over again and then I couldn't get rid of that feeling, over and over and over again. Now I think about it, I might cry but I let it go. So, that sort of stopped a little bit, so I still have the feelings but it doesn't do it over and over and over again.

One of the things that she can still feel unhappy about is that, in comparison to others, she isn't doing as well. She knows, on an intellectual level that everyone is different and that recovery depends on a lot of different factors, including where exactly the brain damage occurred, but she said:

> Sometimes, I get really disgusted hearing that "this friend had an aneurysm and she is now back to work and all." I hate that feeling! That I am *not* doing what I need in order to go back to work and resume my old life. Why is it that some people can do it and other people can't? I know that there are different areas where it is located but still, it sucks! I feel bad, that I am not doing it right as far as rehab and stuff, like there is a secret and I didn't get the answer. I need to stay away from the comparisons.

Regarding her experience of aphasia, she is surprised to find that when she is angry, she can talk easily. While I'm unaware of research on how emotion can affect aphasia, it's something that anecdotally seems not uncommon. For me, anger can be a trigger for my mild aphasia, and I lose my ability to express myself.

Katherine doesn't have difficulty acknowledging that she now has mobility impairments so that it can sometimes be difficult to walk or do things requiring fine motor skills. Yet she is optimistic about continuing recovery in that area. She believes that with exercise, it will be possible to move beyond her current recovery plateau. She is highly motivated to set goals for herself and never to give up trying to reach them.

Acknowledging her cognitive impairments, however is much harder for Katherine. She tends to move back and forth between recognizing that she has aphasia and challenging the label. On the one hand, she knows that she has challenges, but on the other hand, she doesn't like the way using the label of aphasia erases her individuality. Aphasia, she knows, can be manifested quite differently from individual to individual, and she wants her unique situation to be understood. She doesn't want to have her experiences glossed over. For similar reasons, she doesn't like being understood as having a brain injury. For example, though at the time of the interview she was enrolled in a state program for people with brain injury, she has a hard time applying the term to herself. She is comfortable, she said, with talking about having had an aneurysm, or even a stroke, but she shudders when others make reference to her having had a *brain* injury. She doesn't even like to think about the fact that she has had brain surgery. She is not sure why she has such a negative reaction to references to her brain injury, but suspects that it may be because she spent a good part of her pre-stroke life identifying with her cognitive abilities. Now that she is unable to display her abilities so that others will easily recognize her intellect, she feels inferior.

Katherine is similarly troubled with the idea of calling herself disabled:

> Even now, I still have a hard time using the word disability. And, um, let alone brain injury. Let alone aphasia. I think disability is someone in a wheelchair and — you know, it's funny because when I'm on the other side, where I'm a therapist, then I talk about all this and try to convince the clients why it's not the end of the world. But when it's actually happening to *you*, it has changed. And it's just overwhelming. I don't say I'm disabled, because I feel embarrassed. Even when I use the parking placard for the driving I feel like I'm doing something wrong. But then I get annoyed because I can't walk from here to there.

Katherine explained that her embarrassment about being seen as disabled is partly tied to the fact that she is so young yet has such significant impairments. This doesn't fit with her idea about how things should be. She is painfully self-conscious about what she used to be able to do but can no longer do. She was, after all, once the therapist on "the other side" and now she finds herself needing those services herself. There is a sense of shame that goes along with knowing that others look at her and find her deficient or even contemptible. Esther Stein, too, talked explicitly about the humiliation she felt when others saw that she couldn't control her toddler, but most of the other women profiled in this book, including myself, have also felt ashamed at one point or another because we have judged ourselves according to the opinions of others and we have been found wanting. For Katherine, then, the very words "brain injury" or "disability" evoke those feelings of deficiency. She would rather not be reminded of her shame.

Katherine is not sure what her future holds, but she is determined that it will be bright. In her ideal future, she would be living away from her parents. "I'd have a store that does arts and crafts … and then I'd do art therapy on its own for kids. Travel. Hang out with my friends," she told me.

For now, it is one day at a time. She is not sure that she'll ever be able to do art therapy with kids again, but she knows that amazing things can happen with the right therapy. She gets angry when people tell her that she will never be able to do something, because she has seen her own improvements extend beyond the expectations of others, and she has learned of others who have pushed beyond the expectations of professionals. So, she is continually putting herself in places where she can converse with others, and she is continually pushing herself to improve her cognitive skills.

At the same time, she is learning to be kinder to herself. She tries not to get mad at herself when she can't do something. Rather, she tries to celebrate her accomplishments. Thus, she takes time every year on the anniversary of her stroke to write down and reflect on her accomplishments from the past year. She writes down her goals, both short and long term, and creates new goals for herself. In reviewing what has happened, she is able to see that all of the little steps that she has taken are turning into major accomplishments. Katherine has learned that she needs to live one day at a time, and this is what lets her feel good about what she has done. With this philosophy, she can imagine a better future. It may not come as quickly as she might like, but she knows she will get there. Meanwhile, she is determined to enjoy her life.

*

The loss of one's former level of independence can be among the most difficult things about adapting to the sudden changes brought on by a trauma such as stroke. One is faced with redefining what dependence and independence mean and recognizing that they are in an ever-changing new balance. It is important to note that Katherine was only four-and-a-half years post-stroke when I interviewed her. Other women in this book were also dependent on the care of others four years after their strokes, and it is reasonable to suspect that Katherine, when she is ready, will move away from her parents. For the time being, however — and this is vitally important — Katherine wants to stay with her parents because of the financial security she can have by living with them, as well as the loving attention she receives. It's a strategic self-care choice and a positive one, though her former self equated striking out on her own with independence.

From a certain perspective, it would be easy to read Katherine's story and focus on the overwhelming losses she has endured. From a different perspective, though, we can see Katherine's outgoing, creative nature and her story can be read as inspiring. She is dealing with her depression. She goes out of her way to find the supports that she needs to create a good quality of life for herself. She seeks out the therapies that she knows will help her, and she seeks out the help she needs to pay for them. All signs of agency and independence. She has developed a network of supportive relationships — mostly in cyberspace, but nevertheless important to her sense of well-being. Considering all that she has done since her stroke, loss hardly seems an appropriate term for summing up Katherine's experience. I would venture to guess that she will go far in her life.

Vicky Evans

THE IMPORTANCE OF FEELING GENUINE:
CAREER AND IDENTITY

In 1997, when Vicky Evans was thirty-one, she had an intra-cerebral hemorrhage. A couple of years later, I read a newspaper article about the therapeutic benefits of pets that featured Vicky, and I tracked her down to ask if I could interview her. In 2000, I drove out to her home in the countryside east of Toronto — an old farmhouse that had been renovated. I was greeted effusively first by her two dogs and then by Vicky herself. We went into her large kitchen to talk, with occasional interruptions from her three curious cats. Being only three years post-stroke, Vicky was much closer in time than some of the women in the preceding stories to the trauma of the experience. Yet it became clear that she had spent a lot of time thinking about the impact the stroke had had on her life. Vicky, who is of Austrian and English descent, was thirty-four at the time of the interview.

In her story, career and work feature as a significant theme. She repeatedly returns to talking about the career she once had and how her thoughts about career and work have changed since her stroke. Vicky's story also speaks to the role of romantic relationships and social life, and the adaptations one must make to cope with invisible impairments.

*

At thirty-one years old, Vicky Evans was pleased with how her life was going. She was in a loving, common-law relationship and she had recently landed a position as communications director at a major publishing house in Toronto. She had grown up in Toronto and had been in the publicity business since she was twenty-two.

> I'd gone from one job to the next and I worked really, really hard. I guess you could say I was or maybe am a workaholic type. I was thirty-one, I was director of communications for this company. Which was great! I figured I could double my salary in two years, a year and a half, at this company, and then be VP of communications somewhere else. You know, I was not doing bad for not having a university education [laughing]! And quite, you know, proud of myself.

Her work was vitally important to her sense of self. For this reason, she maintained a persona as a vital, friendly, knowledgeable and community-spirited woman. It's not that she wasn't all of these things, it's that it was important to her to project these qualities so that others would recognize them as essential to who she was. She explains:

> I thought that — and, for the most part I was right — a lot of people [pause] liked me and were attracted to me — whether they be male or female — you know, as friends, or partners or whatever because of what I was. And I did a lot of volunteer work in addition to my job. And at one time I hosted a feminist radio show, and so I had all these things [I did]; I volunteered for planned parenthood, I did the radio show, I was moving my way up the ladder in communications. So I felt *that's* what made me dynamic and interesting as opposed to who I am.

It was also important to Vicky that she appear to be indefatigable:

> And so I was working my ass off and if I ate three meals a day I ate them all at my desk, I'd come home at 10:30, 11:00 at night, have at least a glass, maybe two glasses, maybe three glasses of wine just to unwind so that I could go to bed and get up really early and be at the office by 7:30 and do it all over

again. [At first] I would get into the office for 8:00, but there was a woman who I worked with who I was friends with and she'd get into the office before I did [laughing]. So then I'd get into the office for 7:30 and I'd be damned if I left the office before she did! That's sick! But I think that's what the majority of — well, at least in my experience — Toronto is all based on.

Considering the time and energy that Vicky put into developing a name for herself so that she would continue to move up the corporate ladder, it's amazing that she was able to simultaneously maintain a common-law relationship with Calvin. It worked, though, because Calvin had his own high-powered job to focus on, and both of them agreed to keep the weekends reserved to spend time together as a couple.

Vicky had met Calvin when she was twenty-five, and they moved in together four years later. By November 1997, they had been living together for a year and a half and were preparing to celebrate Christmas for the first time in the house they had recently bought. Vicky, who had fond memories of family Christmas celebrations, wanted to have a Christmas tree in the living room, but Calvin did not share Vicky's fond memories and did not like the idea of getting a tree. The discussion/argument was still going on when Vicky experienced her stroke.

Vicky went to work on November 27, just as on any other weekday. She had been getting tension headaches over the past few weeks, but they were not bad enough for her to be concerned that anything serious was the matter. That evening, she was scheduled to work late because her employer was hosting a gathering for an out-of-town guest, and Vicky was expected to ensure that everything ran smoothly. She remembers that around 8:00 that evening, she began feeling quite nauseous and out of sorts. She pushed through it, and finally got home around 11:00. Calvin was home and as she began telling him about not feeling well, her entire left side went limp. She had an intracerebral hemorrhage — a stroke.

Semi-conscious, she was rushed to the hospital, where she remembers, upon arrival, being asked all sorts of questions, such as what is the date, what is your name and so on. She remembers getting a CT scan, which she didn't like because she didn't want to stay lying down. She kept trying to get up and several people had to hold her down. She continues:

> And I wasn't allowed to go to the bathroom, which really upset me. They made me pee in a bedpan. Not that I could have gotten off the stretcher if I'd wanted to, with my whole left side paralyzed [said with laughter]! I just remember everybody around me, and it being very confusing. People asking me things and I just wanted to go to sleep. And the doctor — there was a young intern, and she kept on prying my eyelids open with her hands. Ah, I was so angry! And I turned to my mother — 'cause Calvin had called my parents and they were there — I turned to my mother, and I'm saying: "Make her go away! Like, get her away from me! 'Cause I just can't." I didn't like that.

For the first two days in hospital, Vicky was paralyzed on her left side. She recalls being amazed by the constant parade of visitors, as she had not realized just how many people cared about her. About this, she said:

> It's unfortunate that it takes something horrible to find out how much people care about you. But I got flowers, cards, letters from people I hadn't heard from in a while. From people in the media that had heard from another publicist. Oh, you know, publicists are great with gossip: "Oh, did you hear about Vicky?" And they would write me or send me a card, or call me up and say, "Vicky, I'm so sorry. We're all rooting for you!" And it was that that also helped with how I looked at things. You know, that whole idea that [pause] I have made a difference. It may not be on a global scale — 'cause I think we all want to do something special or make a difference somehow. You know, and some people choose to do that through having children, or whatever. But it was like, I've touched people. And in a good way. And that was nice. That was nice to know that people that I hadn't really thought cared enough to take the time out of their busy schedules to give me a shout or whatever [took the time to care].

Then, on the third day in hospital, she was able to move her left thumb. She said:

And you've never seen a room full of people so happy in your life. At seeing the little thumb move! And eventually, slowly, and actually quite rapidly after that as the days progressed, my left side got stronger and I could move it.

After a week in hospital, her doctors thought that she should be discharged to a rehabilitation facility for physical therapy, but there was a waiting list and they decided that she would do better at home. They were very pleased with how she was recovering from the stroke, and kept saying that because of her youth, they expected that she would get better quickly and regain almost all of her physical abilities. It seems unlikely that her youth was the real reason for the optimistic prognosis, given that other women profiled in this book were younger than Vicky but had, in an objective sense, worse outcomes. Rather, it seems likely that Vicky's doctors were encouraged about her ability to recover based on where her hemorrhage had been located and how extensive it was. Nevertheless, Vicky and those around her were satisfied and encouraged by this explanation of her progress.

Interestingly, everyone focused on Vicky's physical impairments. No one suggested that she might have also been left with cognitive impairments, and no one warned her that she might experience debilitating fatigue in the months or years to come. As we will see later in her story, however, she soon became aware of how little it took before she would feel a profound sense of fatigue, and she went on to become aware of subtle differences in her cognition. These were things she only became aware of as she attempted to get on with her life. We can only speculate about why she wasn't warned about these possibilities while she was still in hospital or at a follow-up appointment with a neurologist. Perhaps her doctors wanted to "leave well enough alone," and not worry her about what was not obvious.

Vicky was able to return home because Calvin was able to negotiate with his employer to stay off work for a month and a half, with pay. Vicky knows that she was fortunate to have Calvin willing to act as her full-time nurse and her mother as back-up, while friends were happy to fill in from time to time. She was touched by how Calvin willingly took charge of caring for her, and she saw this as evidence of the depth of his commitment to her:

> We'd lived together a year and a half at that point. And, you know, you don't often get as lucky as I did. He's pretty incredible. I really tested him and our relationship. He came through for me and I don't know if the shoe had been on the other foot if I would have been as good as he was.

As it was, Calvin could not do enough to show her how much he cared. When Vicky got home from hospital, Calvin made sure there was a Christmas tree waiting for her.

Although Vicky was regaining more and more use of her left side daily, she was nevertheless not able to walk very well or do much for herself for quite a while after getting home. She was very rarely left on her own, as everyone was afraid that she would fall or otherwise hurt herself. She said:

> I was banned from going upstairs [laughing]! I was given strict rules if I was home alone: "You're not allowed to go upstairs. You're not allowed to shower or bake on you own." 'Cause I'm sure everybody thought that I was going to fall and drown. So, my secret pleasure was going up the stairs by myself [laughing]! I wouldn't take a bath or a shower 'cause that kind of scared me. But I would attempt to go up and down the stairs by myself because it was important to me to be able to do that.

Once Vicky had been home for a while, she felt she needed something to focus on other than simply recovery, and she wanted to feel that she was contributing towards her and Calvin's well-being. She decided that the way to do this was to learn how to cook. She hasn't, she says, become "a culinary goddess," but at the time, it was important to her to be able to say to Calvin when he came from work, "Today I made macaroni and cheese for the very first time."

On one hand, Vicky felt infantilized by all the attention she got when she first came home from the hospital, and to a certain extent, was continuing to get at the time of the interview:

> I felt like a little kid again. It really infantilizes you. And one of the lasting effects, not for me but for those who love me, is that

when I stay out here [in the country] by myself — if Calvin has to work in Calgary, or Vancouver or wherever, or he stays in the city — I get lots of phone calls: "Well you sure you're okay?" You know? I never think twice about it. But everybody who cares about me does. It's interesting, you know, they still worry. I think it's much scarier for them than it is for me, you know?

On the other hand, she said:

It's kinda weird being treated as a fragile person. Not that it happens as much anymore, but friends still worry about me like I hadn't learned anything. Every once in a while, my mom and dad will say something. Or Calvin will say something. And I used to get angry about it because, you know, I'm thirty-four goddamn it, and I'm independent and I can do this by myself! And how dare you think I can't do it? And now I realize that it's not that, it's just that they're concerned, but sometimes you just go, "When will I no longer be the stroke survivor?" [laughing] You know? When does that end? Is there an anniversary date or something, that people will stop thinking about that?

After she got home from the hospital, it took Vicky about six months before she felt that she had recovered enough on an emotional level to be able to deal with taking charge of situations on her own. For instance, she felt incapable of negotiating what she would do with her doctors, so Calvin did a lot of advocating on her behalf. A number of times she would be on the telephone with her doctors and end up in tears because she just didn't seem to be able to talk to them about what she wanted.

It's not clear why Vicky was having problems taking charge of situations or advocating on her own behalf. She was not aphasic — she had no trouble understanding others or expressing herself — but her difficulties would seem to indicate that her cognitive skills had been impaired. Cognitive skills are generally divided into the areas of attention, memory, visual-spatial skills, language and executive function. The latter area includes high-level skills such as planning and preparing for activity and this is what was difficult for Vicky. At this stage, however, it did not occur to her to wonder about possible impairment of her cognitive skills. Rather, she assumed that her problems stemmed from the shock of her stroke and that she was still feeling so emotionally vulnerable.

Her vulnerability led to changes in her relationship with Calvin. She came to see him in a new light:

> It changed our relationship, for the better. Not that it wasn't a good relationship to begin with. But I think it made it deeper. It made me realize, it made me realize what — that whole idea of forever? You know? I'd never really understood it. Like I'd always taken for granted that we were together but I knew that it still could very well fall apart. Anything's possible. But I never really appreciated that whole idea of loving forever until I was sick.

The stroke affected Vicky's left side. After she got home, she had physical therapy (paid for by health insurance), although she has little to say about this. For Vicky, the difficulties that went along with the left-sided weakness were (and remain) "more like a nuisance." Even so, "they were a daily reminder that this is what had happened." She elaborates:

> I would drag my left foot and I still do when I'm tired. I hold my arm bent, close to my body. And it's negligible, but these two fingers are not — I tend to keep my fist clenched all the time. And I don't use them. I'm really awful that way. I have to try and force myself to use all of my fingers. And when I'm tired, I don't pick up my left foot. And I fall quite often [laughs]. So I have to consciously focus on what I'm doing.

When she first got home from the hospital, she expected that she would take some time to recover and then return to her career. Vicky said, "I just thought that, well, I'll just get better." So, she got to work on relearning how to walk, how to use her left arm and hand, how to maintain her balance, even how to smile (because, as she says, "that was one of the weird things — my left side didn't smile"). She found, however, that these relatively visible, tangible problems were easy to deal with compared with other, unforeseen obstacles that were a consequence of her stroke:

> What I didn't count on was the exhaustion. And I get it now. If I have a late night I get that "in your bones" tired. And my girl-

friend said to me, "You know, it's just aging." And you know what? This is not age. I can stay up, but if I don't go to bed at a decent hour and get a certain amount of sleep on a consistent basis, then I just drag myself around. I didn't count on the extreme exhaustion I would feel, like the having to have naps all the time. Nor did I [count on depression] — really, I've never been a depressed person. I've always been a fairly introspective person. But I'd always been fairly happy and never imagined that I could be so [pause], I won't say depressed, because I don't know. But, I would cry at anything. And I just felt that I couldn't [pause] move forward sometimes.

The exhaustion and the depression, I guess, well, depression, were overwhelming. And the fact that, you know, you go from being vital — not that you're not still vital, but you're vital in a different way. You know, I did this, and I did this, and I have a job, and I was social, and I had lots of friends. And all of a sudden your world is you, and my animals, and Calvin and his parents. My parents too, but his parents are retired. So, Calvin's mother would come over and do my housework for me and cook meals for us. And you go from having gone everywhere by yourself to now going nowhere alone. And not going anywhere a lot. So, psychologically it's tough. It is a [pause] big thing.

Vicky could have used some psychological counselling to help her cope with her fatigue and depression, but she didn't think to seek out such help, nor did anyone suggest it. Instead, she coped as best she could by relying on the support of her family. It was also important to her that she show her appreciation for their support by, in part, working to take care of traditional housewifely activities such as cleaning and cooking. Vicky did not say whether she took primary responsibility for these things before her stroke, but it is striking to note her mention of taking responsibility for these activities after her stroke. Vicky was feeling inadequate in terms of her inability to bounce right back into her career, and we can wonder whether this was her way, at least at the time, of regaining a sense of self-esteem. Perhaps she wasn't a high-powered media executive, but she at least could take care of her home. This has long been a way for women who are denied access to the public world to hold on to a sense of self-esteem.

Vicky managed to get through the worst of the depression, although she says she still isn't as upbeat or as energetic as she was before the stroke. She said:

> But I'm nowhere near what I was. But, you know, it'll be three years this November, and I look at it and — you know, I remember crying because I was so tired or whatever — and I just think, "This will never be any different. It will never change. I will always be like this." You get to that point where you can't see the end of the tunnel, and think, "This is gonna be it. I'm never gonna get beyond this." And then all of a sudden you're beyond that.

One might expect that being able to go back to work was a key factor allowing Vicky to emerge from her depression, but going back to work actually served to make her feel worse. While Vicky was at home, she was able to be kind to herself. She could feel safe and secure surrounded by those who loved her. She could also fantasize about how wonderful it would be to return to her old life — perhaps with a few adjustments being made — but her old life, nevertheless. The reality of going back to work, though, was that it was scary to be out in public where there were expectations about performance:

> When I started to really get better I went back to work. But I didn't go back to my old job, I went back on contract to do publicity [for a different company]. It was very important for me to go back, to know that I could do it and that people would want to hire me. One of the things that really bothered me was that I couldn't speak well — I had spent twelve years of my life on the phone, and here I had a phobia about talking on the phone because I didn't sound right. So when I first started back I had that still. I felt kind of that I was losing it, like it was all getting all jumbled up. That was something that I was extremely focused on after the stroke, after I started to get back in circulation as it were. I would come home, say to Calvin, "Do I still talk funny?" or "Is my smile back?" You know, constantly

checking to see if I had changed 'cause I wanted so much not to have changed from who I was.

And not that I needed to put on a brave face, but I pushed myself and did things when I was too tired to do them, and tried very hard to not be different. And not give in to the exhaustion or whatever it was. And that worked to my disadvantage. Because then everybody quickly forgot that I had been through something extremely traumatic. You know, I remember being in the washroom one day at work thinking, not a day goes by that I don't remember that I've had a stroke. I notice it either in the way I speak, perhaps in the way I move, or you know, stupid things like toilet paper happens be to on this side [the left side], or getting into a small cubicle in the bathroom.

So then I accepted another job at the same company as the associate artistic director for a festival. It was well, what the hell, you know? It's an adventure. It's something different. And it was — it was exciting and it was interesting.

Vicky was quite happy with her new position: "I was comfortable. People knew me, liked me, I liked them. It was quite wonderful." Her former boss, though, began to plead with her to return to the job she had been doing at the time of the stroke. This did wonders for her battered ego:

I thought no one would want me. You know: "Well, her body failed her once. What's to say it won't happen again? She just doesn't have the stuff. She's not tough enough." And going back to my old employer was important for me because I had to prove to myself that I could do the job. And that I wasn't weak. I thought there was something bad in being weak.

Eventually, Vicky decided to give it a try. She lasted for about four months, and then decided to quit. She came to realize that her experience had changed her on more than a physical level: "I worked really hard at being who I was again and then realized that I will never be that person again. And that's not a bad thing. That's okay." She elaborates:

And when I went back to work I remember thinking, "This is all shit! This doesn't mean anything! We're not doing anything constructive here!" Like, how can I go from such a life-death experience to pedalling entertainment again! You know? And telling people to come to concerts and talking to the media and it was … so much bullshit! I couldn't see me ever wanting to do it ever again, ever putting my heart into it. It just didn't ring true anymore.

I also felt I was trying to prove something to my boss and to the people who worked there when I was there. And I didn't need to prove anything. But I had to figure that out for myself. And I went there and I thought: "These people are sick [laughs]! I don't like this. I don't need to do this. I don't — this is not important to me!" And so then I quit out of my own volition.

Vicky is no longer interested in having a career in publicity. As she said, "There's no way I can do publicity ever again. I just don't feel genuine." She finds that even though she has recovered to the point that no one would notice anything different about her, she no longer has the physical stamina that she had before. Once she came to terms with that, she began to feel better about herself.

Since quitting her last job, Vicky has been content to work with the occasional short-term contract, while remaining unemployed between jobs. A few months before I interviewed her, she had spent three weeks acting as the media liaison for a festival. She approached the job quite differently, though, than she might have approached it even a year earlier. She said:

> You know, Calvin was really worried when I went and worked on the festival for three weeks. But he's starting more and more to realize that I'm not the same person I was before. At the festival I would leave a party or not go to the party and go to bed early. Or people would go out partying and I'd really want to be part of it, but I'd realize that if I did, the next day I wouldn't be functional. So, I'd go back to my hotel room for 9:00 or whatever, and go straight to bed. Or I'd go to a reception and I wouldn't drink. I can't do those things anymore. And now I listen to my body.

Vicky also pointed out that going to parties, mixing with lots of people and generally being seen as friendly were all important parts of being in the publicity business. But, even if she did not find that parties began too late in the day for her, she found that she had become uncomfortable at parties. She said, "I haven't told anybody that I don't feel comfortable in those kinds of situations. I've told Calvin, but I don't think people really fully understand it."

Although Vicky did not talk in terms of cognitive impairment, she experienced changes in her ability to process information. As is so often the case, though, her cognitive impairment is extremely subtle — so subtle that she herself wonders whether her difficulties are due to the residual effects of her stroke or something else. At first, she said, she thought that her lack of comfort in social situations was because she had been "out of circulation" for so long. Over time, though, she began to realize that this was not the problem; she could no longer cope with any situation involving more than a few people. She found them disorienting.

Her comfort level changed post-stroke in part because of physical difficulties with managing the logistics of circulating at parties ("I find if I hold my glass with my right hand then I can't shake with my left hand [laughing]. And then I don't feel comfortable holding the glass with my left hand, because I have a tendency when I talk to tip it"), but more importantly, because of new difficulties with taking in a lot of information at once:

> Before I used to be able to have a couple of conversations at once and now I just can't. I find I need to do one-on-one or a couple of people. I find big dinner parties really not a lot of fun anymore, either. I just find it very — well, I can't focus … It's not that I'm distracted easily, it's just that I find that there's just too many points of stimulation. It's overwhelming. I have a great feeling of there being just too much going on. I guess it's overstimulation.

There are striking similarities between what Vicky said about her sense of being overstimulated and what Lauren Mayes said about feeling overwhelmed in busy environments. Both women had strokes in the right hemisphere of the brain (each hemisphere controls the opposite side of the body, thus a right-hemisphere stroke affects the left side of the body). Vicky's hemorrhage does not appear to have been as extensive as Lauren's was, yet it is amazing to find that Vicky repeated, almost word for word, what Lauren said about her lasting cognitive impairments. Even more amazing, though, is that Vicky's stroke was almost thirty years after Lauren's. Despite the knowledge that has accumulated since then, there was still no one to explain to Vicky that she might experience cognitive difficulties, and there was no one to help her figure out how to deal with those difficulties.

Vicky's new lack of comfort in large groups of people means that she has a vastly constrained social life. These days, it's all she can do to cope with family gatherings. Her world has essentially shrunk, as she said, to her animals, her partner and his parents. Before the stroke, she thrived on living in a large, cosmopolitan city with an abundance of cultural and entertainment venues. Since the stroke, though, she sees few people socially.

To some extent, Vicky's reluctance to participate in large gatherings played a part in her and Calvin's decision, two years after her stroke, to move from the city to a house in the country, several hours away. She and Calvin, she said, were no longer "using the city as much as we were before." When she told her friends about their decision to move, they protested:

"Well, you're gonna miss such-and-such, and such-and-such." And it was like, "We never go out [laughing]!" You know, we were in the city and we stayed at our house all week. We never went anywhere, so how can you miss something you don't do anymore?

She has discovered a part of herself "that *loves* not being in touch" with what's going on in the city. She goes into the city infrequently, and when she goes, she tends to be concerned about appearing "naive or ignorant," but she recognizes that:

I don't need to know all those things. I probably didn't need to know them to begin with. I felt that I did, though. It's also that whole who you are and who you know and what you know, which is really important in the industry that I was in. And now I know that it's enough to be who I am and that if that's not enough for them, then forget it.

Even though Vicky has lost interest in working as a publicist, she nevertheless realized early on that her professional skills and contacts put her in a good position to raise awareness about stroke. She knew that her own stroke was precipitated by uncontrolled high blood pressure, and she wanted to warn others to take high blood pressure more seriously than she did. She decided to volunteer for the Heart & Stroke Foundation, and for two years she served as a media spokesperson. She said it was "one of the best things I ever did after having the stroke," and "I get just as much if not more out of it than other people get. I've found talking about it very therapeutic."

There are aspects of her experience, however, that Vicky feels she can only talk about with a select few, because she does not want her concerns dismissed as trivial:

> You can't really got to your doctor and say, "You know what? I'm uncomfortable at a cocktail party." "So?" That's a really big deal, you know? [laughing] Or, "These two fingers don't work well. I don't type well." And, "Whippy-ding-dong! You have use of both of your hands."

Vicky is interested in knowing that she is not alone in her experiences; that others have had similar experiences. She is also somewhat surprised to find herself wanting this, because, she explains, "I always wanted to be an individual. So it's kind of funny for someone like me who worked so hard to be different and to be an individual. There are parts of me now that look for commonality in other people."

From the vantage point of almost three years post-stroke, Vicky is able to make a statement that many people might find incredible. "No one needs to say, 'Poor Vicky,' or, 'What a horrible thing.' 'Cause it wasn't. It's actually been one of the best things that's ever happened to me. Ironically."

She feels this way because of all she has learned from her experience. She has learned, in particular, that she needed to change her approach to life — that life is not a competition to be rushed through. When friends suggest to her that she had the stroke because the demands of her job were too high, she counters that the demands of the job were not unreasonable. Rather, she says: "It was how I chose to approach it and now I'll never work for anyone that hard again, 'cause no one is worth it. No one."

Before her stroke, Vicky lived mostly for the future. She was not focused on enjoying the present. Someone asked her, at one point, whether she had been happy in the three months she worked at the publishing house before the stroke. She said:

> I didn't have time to ask myself, "Are you happy?" I was just doing it. And thinking, "Okay, if I put in a good year, maybe a year and a half, then I can jump to some other company and it'll all be worth it [laughing]." So it almost killed me [laughing]!

She has learned to rejoice in what she has, rather than worry about what she does not have:

> I feel like I've been given an opportunity to appreciate life more. And I think that — I'm getting teary — it just means more to me now. And I've now realized that it's okay to be just me. That I don't need to be director of communications. That I don't need to make x-amount of thousands of dollars a year. That it's enough to love my animals and Calvin.
>
> I think that one thing that did come out of the stroke, that I never used to do before, is I was a great planner in that, you know, when I do this, or I will do this, I will be this in such and such. Set a time, or whatever. And now it's day to day. I make plans. I'd like my garden to be like this next year. But I don't know if we'll be here. You know, it's one day at a time, which I never really did before. I lived a lot in the future, and I think that's one of the bad things about society, is we live too much in the future or in the past. And we don't live for now. And I think that *that* out of everything is one of the biggest and best things that I've gotten from my experience: that it's today, you know?

*

Vicky has moved from being almost entirely focused on climbing the corporate hierarchy in her career to learning to appreciate the joy of simply *being*. She is explicitly thankful that she was able to learn this lesson at a relatively young age. Along the way, she did not get the best rehabilitation, but she had a great deal of support from friends and loved ones, so she never had to face her difficulties entirely alone. Her impairments are invisible to others, and this makes it hard for her to talk about them to both friends and physicians. She has become determined, nevertheless, not to let her impairments get in the way of enjoying her life. That it took a life-threatening stroke for Vicky to learn how to slow down might, in one sense, seem sad, but in another sense, it is important that we join Vicky in acknowledging that life goes on and is definitely to be celebrated in the here and now.

Cindy Davis

The Best Thing that Ever Happened:
Attitude and Acceptance

Cindy Davis, a woman of English and Irish descent, was forty-two years old when we met in late 2002. In 1998, when she was thirty-eight, she had a subarachnoid hemorrhage due to a ruptured aneurysm. Cindy lives in a remote village near the town of Redruth in Cornwall, on the west coast of England. Before we settled down to begin the interview, Cindy took great pride in showing me her small house, which she loved, and she was especially pleased with the view of the sea afforded from one of her windows. Then we went into her living room to talk, joined by her two cats.

There are a number of themes in Cindy's story that also appear in the stories of other women. These include career and work, financial resources and invisible impairment. Woven throughout her story, however, I see the overarching themes of attitude and acceptance. Of all the women in this book, Cindy stands out in terms of the optimism with which she has faced her post-stroke life and the way in which she has so quickly come to accept that her impairments are now simply a part of life — no more and no less.

*

In August 1998, Cindy Davis was living in Buckinghamshire, England. At thirty-eight, she had already experienced a number of losses and traumas. Her father had died of cancer in 1986, when she was twenty-six. Her mother developed breast cancer and had a mastectomy in 1997; she seemed to be doing well after that, but there was always the threat of its return. Then in July of 1998, Cindy's aunt, who had been in a nursing home, died of pneumonia. Cindy was responsible for putting her aunt's affairs in order — sorting out her funeral, her will and all her belongings — and she found that very stressful. She was also coping with the aftermath of her second divorce, which had taken place in 1997. Cindy had moved in with her seventy-eight-year-old mother after the divorce, and all was going nicely there, but it was nevertheless stressful for Cindy to be living with her mother, who was not dealing well with her sister's death. Cindy was still reeling from the trauma of yet another marriage breakdown. She felt that she needed a man in her life, and she was in the process of searching for husband number three. She was able to cope with all these pressures because she had a strong group of friends and she maintained an active social life.

Cindy had a degree in psychology and then she decided that she wanted to be a nurse, as her mother was. After a few false starts towards completing her training to become a registered nurse, she finished and got a job as a nurse. After eighteen months, though, she decided that she didn't like the work after all. She started looking for something else to do, and in 1998 she landed a job to train as a medical researcher. The new job involved travelling to interview nurses, doctors and patients. She found it quite interesting and exciting, and an added bonus was that she got "a great company car, a Golf GTI that was wonderful!" She was looking forward to moving up in the organization. Yet she was also "under loads and loads of pressure" at work.

In late July, Cindy went to her doctor because she had had a headache for a week. She was used to getting headaches, having been plagued with them as far back as she could remember. Once every few months she would get a "*huge*" headache that would last most of the day and be incapacitating. These headaches did go away. This one, though, was different. Her doctor more or less dismissed her concerns, telling her that her headache was not surprising, considering how much stress she had been under lately. It's not clear why her doctor downplayed her concern about the unusual headache, but we can speculate that he might not have so readily sent a male patient home with no further investigation. Nevertheless, Cindy was satisfied with the diagnosis. She thought to herself, "that's fair enough," and she went home again.

A few days later, on August 2, 1998, Cindy was in the bathroom at home when she collapsed. She doesn't remember what happened for eight weeks after that. She must have made a noise, though, as her mother came in to find her unconscious on the floor. Her mother had to break in, because Cindy had locked the bathroom door. Her mother immediately called an ambulance and accompanied Cindy to the local hospital where she had trained as a nurse.

The doctors assessed Cindy, who was unconscious, and for reasons unknown to Cindy decided that she had a urinary tract infection. She was given some antibiotics and told to go home. Her mother was not willing to accept that diagnosis, though, and insisted that Cindy be evaluated further. Cindy stayed at the hospital's Accident and Emergency for another ten hours, at which point one of her pupils became markedly dilated, and she began vomiting. These signs of neurological problems got the doctors' attention and she was whisked off for a CT scan. The scan showed that her brain had hemorrhaged, and she was immediately prepared for transfer to a larger hospital with a sophisticated neurological unit.

The next day, Cindy had surgery to clip her ruptured aneurysm, and because she was not returning to consciousness as expected and she was not breathing well, she was put on a ventilator for ten days. She developed hydrocephalus and had to have a second surgery to insert a ventriculo-peritoneal shunt that would drain excess fluid from her brain. After that, she started to improve. Still, it was another several weeks before Cindy became stable enough to be moved out of the intensive care unit, and she remained mostly unconscious.

Aside from one incident she had while still on the ventilator in the ICU, Cindy remembers nothing from the time she spent at the larger hospital:

> I had this weird experience with all these energies, and one of those energies was my dad, who'd died in eighty-six. And the other one was the aunt who'd died the week before [her stroke]. And they basically told me I shouldn't be going with them. I needed to go back and look after my mom. So they sent me back. And back I went, and thought, "Oh! Okay then."

Cindy did not elaborate on the sense she made of this experience, beyond saying that she took it as a message that she wasn't going to die — that she still had work to do on earth. At a later point in the interview, however, she commented on her spiritual beliefs, saying: "But I *do* believe that when I die, I'm going to go on somewhere else. Because that's what I saw when I had my experience."

Cindy had been a church-going Anglican before her stroke, although she said that she never fully believed all that the church taught. Since the stroke, however, she told me that she had developed a strong belief in angels and had an angel in her garden who was looking after the garden for her. That experience in the hospital was spiritually very important for her, even empowering; it perhaps provided an important motivation for her to recover and go on to reshape her life.

After eight weeks, she was moved back to her local hospital where she received physical, occupational and speech therapy. She can remember bits and pieces of her stay there, although she wasn't entirely oriented to what was going on around her. For instance, she would forget that she had become paralyzed on her right side. She remembers doing "silly things" such as sitting on the toilet and not having the sense to ring for help when she wanted to get up. She wasn't able to get up by herself, so she would just sit there until someone came: "I couldn't walk, I couldn't move my arm, couldn't do anything. Fortunately I'm left-handed, so I could still write and do all that kind of thing."

She also remembers getting lots of visits from friends. She said:

> I had so many cards and stuff when I was in hospital, and presents, and I've still got teddies and stuff that everyone gave me [laugh]. They used to come and check up on me, used to come and see me, take me out, which was fun. And they're still there, all of them.

Cindy spent three weeks at her local hospital, receiving help from "lots of therapists." She was fortunate to have private health insurance through her employer, so she feels that she got better rehabilitation services than she would have received had she been without insurance. Without insurance, she would have had to stay in a ward of the National Health Service — the government-run health care provider in the UK — and she is not sure that she would have received as much therapy. Nevertheless, she was anxious to leave the hospital as soon as she could:

> I just wanted to go home. I just needed to go home because I knew I'd be okay when I went home. *I WAS NOT OK IN THAT PLACE!* You know, they were interrupting me all the time, they were coming in, bothering me about this, that and the other and I wasn't getting any peace and *I NEEDED PEACE.* Actually, I think I was quite stressed by being there. Thinking back, I remember I desperately wanted to go home, and I saw this occupational therapist who said, "Right, I'm going to take you home for a visit. You can go home and see the cats and your mom." So, they took me home and I needed to prove to them that I'd be okay there. My mom had really steep stairs, but there were banisters on both sides so it was easy. I could get up the stairs. I went in and I said, "Right, I'm going to prove it," and I went up these stairs and came back down them and said, "See? See? I can come out!"

Shortly after that, Cindy's doctors agreed that she would be all right, and they discharged her into her mother's care.

Part of the reason Cindy wanted to go home was because she missed her cats, whom she regarded as family. Also, she hadn't been able to get enough sleep at the hospital, and she desperately wanted to be able to have a good sleep. So, that's the first thing she did when she got home. It's interesting that so many women in this book spoke about not being able to get sleep in the hospital, and then going home to do little else but sleep. In Cindy's case, she said:

> I used to go to bed about nine every night and I used to get up about ten or eleven in the morning. I used to sleep right the way through. No problem! And I slept and slept for about two or three weeks like that. Just sleep. Loads and loads of sleep. And it worked! I started to get better.

Cindy continued physiotherapy and speech therapy as an out-patient, and she also devised her own way of training her right hand to become useful again. She had a computer at home that she liked to use, and even though she was left-handed she had always used the mouse with her right hand. So, she decided to practise using the mouse by playing solitaire on the computer: "I thought if I do solitaire using this mouse and using my right hand, it'll give me strength in my right hand. And it worked! I spent ages doing solitaire, I was so slow at it to start with."

Three months later, in January 1999, Cindy went back to work on a part-time basis. She was walking well, although she had a slight limp when tired, and her right arm was reasonably functional though not very strong. She wasn't able to return to interviewing people, however, because she found that she couldn't say what she wanted to say. At the time, Cindy was not sure why she was having this problem. Nevertheless, her employers were good to her and put her to work with administrative duties. She worked on the computer, something she was good at. After a while, though, her employers weren't happy with the way things were working out, and that October they gave her the option of either moving to the London office or being let go.

Cindy didn't have to think very hard before she decided that she would take the option of leaving her employer. Her mother's cancer had returned in January and she had become quite sick; she died in September 1999, a little more than a year after Cindy's stroke. Cindy had been caring for her mother because there were no relatives around to help. Her mother's death left her bereft of family.

After her mother's death, Cindy decided that she didn't want to stay where she was. Her mother had left her a small legacy, which Cindy used to make a radical break from the past. Barely a month after her mother's death, she started house hunting in a small Cornish village far from the hustle and bustle of southeast England. Inside of three days she looked at fourteen houses, and then she saw a house that she fell in love with. She immediately made an offer to buy the house outright, and in January 2000, she moved in to start a new life. Once she was settled, she set about getting to know the local people:

> I'd been here about three or four months and I went down to the village and said, "Would you like someone to work in your shop?" And the chap there said, "Yes please." So I did like twenty hours a week and I got to know all the locals. So now when I go down into the village — there's about a thousand of us I suppose — I always see someone I know, always have a chat with somebody. Also, there's a sort of tea-room restaurant that I've been going to since I came here and I've become friendly with the people that own it. I'm quite the friendly little soul, really!

As well, she joined a singles club, more to find people to socialize with than to find a new partner. Her stroke has not changed her outgoing and social nature, and she makes friends easily. She quite enjoys going on outings with her new friends:

> There's about thirty of us I suppose, but most events there's maybe five or six will go, and we do all sorts of things. We go bowling, we go to the cinema. I know all the restaurants in this part of the country, all the good ones. And all the good pubs. I've got two *really* close friends from that group and I've also got several who are sort of good mates.

Cindy had by that point lost her desire for yet another boyfriend or husband. She said that her stroke has "taken away my sex urge [laughter], which has been *really* nice!" She was very happy to be on her own: "Since I've had that hemorrhage, I don't need a new husband. I'm very happy on my own, thank you. I don't want one! And that is *completely* the opposite of what I used to be like."

Very little has ever been written regarding sexual desire post-stroke, and there is certainly nothing about the sexuality of young and female stroke survivors. Sexual desire remains a taboo topic, particularly within the context of disability. Cindy, in fact, was one of only two stroke survivors I have ever met who even mentioned sexual desire (the other, who told me of becoming "sex mad" since her stroke, is not profiled in this book). For others, it was not a topic of conversation. In the absence of much "objective" evidence, it is nevertheless worth commenting that there is no reason to suspect that stroke necessarily leaves anyone with a reduced libido. In Cindy's case, it seems likely that her lack of sexual desire is tied to her changed self-image. Since her stroke, she has become much clearer about what she wants out of life, and she has developed the self-confidence to know that she doesn't need a man to feel complete.

Although Cindy was able to recover much of the use of her right side in a relatively short time, she continues to have significant right-sided weakness, which is worse when she's tired. Undaunted, she decided to make exercise a regular part of her new life and joined a gym. Her initial motivation was to shed the extra weight that she had put on after her hospitalization, but she found that the exercises she was doing helped to improve the strength on her right side. This, in turn, helped her with co-ordination.

Her difficulties with using her right side did not stop her from going out to find full-time work that paid a decent wage. After working at the village shop for a while she became quite bored, and she found an entry-level administrative job working at a college in a nearby city. She was very excited to get the job and thought to herself, "*Yes*! I'm on the right route now, I'm getting there!"

Back at work in a demanding job, it became increasingly clear to Cindy that something was wrong with her memory and language skills. Her new job involved going out to lecture halls to set up what was needed to teach courses. She began to feel stressed again, and soon felt that she wasn't able to cope with it. When stressed, she was unable to speak coherently and her memory became so bad that she could forget her own name. She said:

> I didn't realize at that stage, and nobody had ever told me this, that I can't deal with any stress. *Any* stress. And of course, this job was *really, really* stressful. I did it for about three months and my memory had gone, I just couldn't deal with it at all. I used to set everything up for the course and do administration to the lecturers and that kind of thing. I would rush about setting up all these halls and stuff like that.

Her new employer saw that she was struggling and suggested that perhaps she would benefit from some bereavement counselling, considering all that she had been through. So she got in touch with a non-profit organization that offers counselling free of charge. A counsellor came to see Cindy once a week for four or five weeks. They spent an hour each time talking about all her bereavements (not just the consequences of her stroke, but also the deaths of her parents and her aunt, and her divorces) and, at the end of it, Cindy was feeling that she had done well in coming to terms with her losses. Yet she was still having trouble coping with her new job.

After three months of work, Cindy became sick. Her doctor arranged for her to see a rehabilitation consultant. When Cindy saw her and told her about her problems coping with her job, the consultant told her, "You shouldn't be doing that job, you shouldn't be working in *any* stress." This consultant was the first professional to suggest to Cindy that there might be neurological reasons for her difficulties. This information was a revelation to Cindy, and she wondered why no one had ever told her that before. The consultant set in motion arrangements to have Cindy see a neuropsychologist for assessment and cognitive exercises.

Thus, Cindy left her college job and was very happy to do so. She began to feel hopeful that a neuropsychologist could help her with her memory and language skills. Her cognitive difficulties were not really apparent to others, but *she* knew that something was off. She had once had a photographic memory, for example, but that ability was gone. One thing that particularly angered her was that others did not acknowledge the difficulties she now had. She said:

> Because I don't walk with a stick, because I'm able to speak, and because I'm intelligent and therefore can articulate most of what I want to say, so when I say I have problems with language, people say, "Well, you can speak *fine*." "No, I *can't*." *I* know I can't do what I used to be able to do. It's like banging your head against a wall, that. 'Cause, *yes*, people don't recognize that I've got problems.

Getting to actually see a neuropsychologist, however, was easier said than done. Her doctor tried to set up an appointment for her, but found that there was not one neuropsychologist in that part of the country. "So," she said, "I couldn't have an appointment with a neuropsychologist because one didn't exist!"

Unwilling to accept defeat, Cindy persisted in asking her doctor to find a neuropsychologist elsewhere that she could see. Finally, in early 2002, he found one for her and tried to set up an appointment. A month later, Cindy got a letter from the neuropsychologist to say that there was a very long waiting list and she wouldn't be able to get an appointment for years. Cindy then went back to her doctor to complain that she'd already been living with her problems for almost four years, and she shouldn't have to wait another four years. Her doctor got in touch with the neuropsychologist to plead Cindy's case. His intervention worked, and Cindy got an appointment.

By December 2002, when we spoke, Cindy had seen the neuropsychologist twice. She was still in the process of being assessed, but expected that to be finished soon. Already she had been given a few pointers to help her deal with her poor memory:

> It's been *really* beneficial. I wish I'd had it done *years* ago. That is *so* annoying! 'Cause I've been tripping over everything I say, and there might've been something I could *do*. I write everything down, I have to. All my friends now are used to reminding me about everything. And so I've got all these crutches. I've got a to-do list in there, which is great long. *Absolutely* everything I

think needs doing, I have to write it down just to be certain. Some things stick, the big things stick. I remembered you were coming, for example. Which is useful. 'Cause you would have been *really* fed up if you came with no one here!

Cindy expected that after the assessment was completed, she would see the neuropsychologist once more to learn ways of dealing with her memory and speech difficulties. She said: "I think she'll just tell me what to do and then I'll go off and do it. So I don't think I'm going to be going to see her for ages or anything like that. I think it's more to sort of point me in the right direction and send me off."

Getting a diagnosis that pointed to neurological damage served to help Cindy find new ways of working around her cognitive difficulties, and it also allowed her to gain access to the Guide Project, a program for those who have acquired disabilities in adulthood. The program was offered through the college where Cindy had worked and was designed to help people find employment. Cindy was accepted into the program and was able to take several courses to develop her multimedia skills. She very much enjoyed learning these new skills and, based on what she learned, she was able to start her own business teaching computer skills.

When we met, Cindy was excited about the progress she had made in terms of getting clients for her new business, and she was looking forward to expanding her client base. She absolutely loved what she was doing. She had always been "computer mad" and had learned so many new skills through taking courses. Recently, she took up playing with digital photography. She said:

> I teach people one-to-one how to use computers in their homes. That's part of it. Mostly older people, you know, they've got their first-ever computer and they don't know how to use it. So I'll show them. I also mess with images, you know, if they've got photos that need bringing back to life, if they're covered in scratches and stuff like that, I can sort those out. And I do things like newsletters, anything with desktop publishing. I've got my little study and I spend a lot of time in there. I enjoy it.

One of the best things about having her own business is that Cindy's time is her own. She can set her own schedule, deciding what she will or won't do, and when she will or won't work. This greatly reduces the stress that she experiences and leaves time for her to enjoy herself. She loves to travel, and in 2002 went on a one-week trip to Egypt with friends. Her holiday was "*totally incredible,*" but at the same time she was conscious of needing to pace herself so that she would not become exhausted. For example, she would have loved to have joined her friends on a day trip within Egypt, but they were planning to leave at 4:00 in the morning. Cindy knew she wouldn't be able to cope with that, so didn't go. She has learned in the years since her stroke, she said, "to back off and to say no, I can't do this anymore." She doesn't find it in any way depressing to realize that her impairments require her to prioritize her activities and that sometimes things won't get done. In fact, she has never in her post-stroke experiences been depressed. She has generally been too focused on the possibilities open to her to feel unhappy or hopeless.

Cindy has long claimed that "life is not a rehearsal," but this motto has taken on new meaning for her. Before her stroke, she generally interpreted it in terms of the importance of enjoying life. While this has not changed, she has also come to appreciate the importance of being true to herself. Indeed, her personality has changed quite dramatically. She explained:

> I used to be quite submissive and now I'm not. I'm a strappy bugger, I really am. You know, if necessary, I *will* tell people what I think. For instance, I went to a concert in a tavern recently. Really interesting, but the blooming woman in front of me, she just kept standing up! And at the end of it I just went and had a word with her. I said, "*DO YOU REALIZE* that none of us behind you could see anything because you kept standing up?" But I wouldn't have done that four years ago, I'd have just toddled off. But now I'll say something. If somebody jumps the queue or whatever, I'm there. Before, I'd have just put up with it and sulked and looked miserable.
>
> I think because I nearly died — life is not a rehearsal and I need to enjoy it. And now I've become *me*. 'Cause I used to

— when somebody told me what to do I just did it. Now I don't. I just believe that I need to do what *I* want to do, which is why I'm happy on my own. Now as far as I'm concerned I'm blooming perfect so I don't need anybody else [laughter]! In some ways, it was the best thing that ever happened to me. It made me stop and think about myself. And my life and what's important to my life. It's given me direction. It's allowed me to think about life and all that *deep* stuff. And the few disabilities that I've got, I've got used to them now and I'm stuck with them.

Reflecting further on the changes in her life, Cindy also commented that that since her brain hemorrhage, she feels that someone has been looking after her. The feeling stems from the spiritual experience she had in ICU. She certainly feels that there was more than a simple whim to her moving to a house in a distant part of the country:

> I saw this place and I thought, well, that's *it*. I just got the feeling it would work itself out, I felt I was pushed here. I don't think I decided on my own, I think I was told to come here. So, I'm not sure whether I was pushed or pulled [laugh] but I was *made* to come here. And I mean, it was the right move. If I look out there, out of my kitchen and my conservatory, I can see the sea. That's fine. I love it down here. Absolutely wonderful! I think I was looked after. And I think I was helped to get this place, to come here. And life seems to have gone very well since I've been here. You know, I wouldn't be *here*, I wouldn't be in this house, if I hadn't had [the stroke]. Well, maybe I would have, but maybe not for another ten years.

If she had not had the brain hemorrhage, Cindy suspects she'd be "a really posh research exec" and that she'd be "working [her] way through men." "Basically discontented but happy, you know?" She explains:

> But now it's different. Completely different. And it's better. It definitely is better. I'm checking out new experiences and doing things that I've never done before. Going to places I've never been to before. You know, Egypt was a place I was really interested in when I was a kid. When I went there, it was just,

Oh wow, this is wonderful, I'm here! I took 500 photos when I went there. Digital ones, but 500! Life is for living. You have to go out and grab it by the throat.

*

With Cindy's story, we have a particularly vivid example of a woman who was able, in a relatively short period of time, to manifest an enthusiastic determination to live life to the fullest. In this regard, Cindy is a remarkable woman. Adopting a positive and accepting attitude towards surviving stroke and subsequent impairments can be very difficult in a society that sees stroke and impairment as unmitigated tragedy. For most of us, it takes a long time to learn how to see the consequences of stroke in non-mainstream terms, to positively incorporate impairment into a sense of ourselves as a valuable part of who we are and to value our post-stroke lives. Most of us first spend a lot of time grieving, and then we go back and forth between moving towards acceptance and going back to emotional despair, before we are able to get to a place of true acceptance. It is rarely a linear process. Yet it is only when we are able to unequivocally accept our changed realities that we can be said to have truly recovered from stroke. That recovery encompasses far more than simply regaining lost skills. It is a profoundly emotional process.

Since I interviewed Cindy, there have been some noteworthy changes in her life. She continues to live happily in her house by the sea, although she is no longer running her own business. She can't rely on the little that's left of her mother's legacy to support herself and she found that her business would not allow her to make enough money to get by. In 2003, with her characteristic optimism, she set about finding employment elsewhere. She has changed jobs several times since then, but in 2006 was delighted to find work as a representative for a small distribution company. Her job requires driving a small van around the gorgeous scenery in her district to deliver tourist leaflets to various places. She recently told me:

Basically, I go to all the places where the tourists will be going to look for places to visit. I check that all the stands have the right amount of leaflets and stock up. It's great fun because I meet lots of new people and drive around the local coast. Another advantage is that I get lots of exercise and therefore am managing to keep the weight I've lost off. I'm also a lot fitter and I've joined a walking group and have been going out with them every week for nearly a year. Life is great!

Ida King

LEARNING TO LAUGH AT YOURSELF:
LIVING WITH IMPAIRMENT

Ida King had a hemorrhagic stroke in 1995, at age thirty-eight. I met her in person in September 2002, when I drove to her home in Louisville, Kentucky. We arranged for me to arrive in the evening, and she graciously invited me to stay at her apartment overnight so that we could do the interview the next morning. Ida told me that she wouldn't be able to be home until after I had arrived, so she left her door unlocked and told me to walk in and make myself at home while waiting for her. So that's what I did. She arrived about an hour later with her son, then eighteen years old. She greeted me with a warm hug and exclaimed, "Well, look at you!" She was amazed to see that I am not visibly disabled (whereas Ida walks with a pronounced limp). She introduced me to her son, Brad. We shook hands and then he promptly disappeared into his room. I wasn't prepared to start the interview that evening, but Ida was eager to tell me her story right away. So we talked for about an hour, getting to know each other, and I told her as much about my own story as she told me about hers. Soon, though, we decided that it was time to call it a night, so Ida made up the pull-out couch for me in the living room. It was not an easy task for her, but she was determined to do it herself and she would not let me help. When that was done, we all went to bed. The next morning, after Brad had left for school, Ida and I sat in her living room for the formal interview. Ida, who is African-American, was forty-five at the time.

As is true for all the women in this book, Ida has a complex story. Themes that permeate her story revolve around faith, the role of support, motherhood, depression and financial resources. Organizing everything is the theme of living with impairment, as impairment has become her constant companion, determining what she can or cannot do and what she will or will not do. Yet Ida's is not essentially a sad story. She has a wonderful sense of humour, and she has done an amazing job of incorporating impairment into her everyday life.

*

In January 1995, Ida King had been married to Joseph for ten years. Like any marriage, hers had had its ups and downs, but overall it was a good marriage. She and Joseph were close. They typically shared their feelings with each other, supported each other through difficult times (such as the death of Joseph's father) and enjoyed each other's company. They lived in Ida's childhood home with their eleven-year-old son, Brad. She was enmeshed within a web of extended family relations that included her mother, aunts and uncles, and she had a large network of friends from her church. When she wasn't busy with her family, friends or church, she worked as a bookkeeper and assistant office manager for a small business. Her year of studying business administration at college had been put to good use.

Family was important to Ida, so when she saw that her mother and aunt were having trouble caring for her favourite uncle, who had lost a leg due to diabetes, she asked her uncle to move in with her, Joseph and Brad, so that she could oversee his care. She willingly took over this caregiver role, feeling that it was her duty. However, her life was about to change radically.

One evening Ida and Joseph were making love when, suddenly, Ida had a stroke:

> I felt like somebody just knocked me off the bed because what I did was I fell off the bed. And we had a queen size bed and my side of the bed was over against the wall — so when it knocked me over, I fell between the wall and the bed. And I had a foot-board in there, but it had a tall thing on the end of it and when I fell, I didn't fall *on* the floor, but I was wedged between the bed and the wall. And I didn't know what was going on, I was wondering, what's wrong? You know. And my husband got out of bed and he came around … to the foot of the bed where I was wedged in between the wall and stuff, and he kept asking, "What's wrong? What's wrong?" And I told him, "Well, just help me up," and it seemed like all I needed was for him to help me up because I couldn't get up — and see, I didn't know what was happening.
>
> And then the next thing I remember was the firemen were there. I guess he called 911, and they came and they helped me get up; they got me up and laid me on the bed, and they had wrapped me in I guess the bedspread or whatever. So they had to carry me from the back bedroom in this bedspread up to the gurney and they put me on the gurney. I remember that much, and I really don't remember too much else. I remember that they carried me down my front steps and I remember looking up at the sky 'cause I remember seeing the stars in the sky. And then I don't remember anything.

Ida was taken to University Hospital, but she remembers nothing about this. She was quickly diagnosed as having had a stroke, and spent the next few weeks in intensive care, drifting in and out of consciousness. At one point she was moved to a regular room in a ward, but she was quickly taken back to intensive care because her blood pressure was extremely high and she needed to be monitored closely. Mostly she is only able to piece together what happened over the next few weeks by relying on what others have told her. She explained, "I went back up to the hospital one time and the guy looked at me, he said, 'I remember you. When they brought you in, you was sick, you were bad off, they didn't think you was gonna make it.'"

Many friends and family visited her, but she can recall only a few. She feels badly about not remembering those who came:

> My mother and her sister, they were there every day, but I don't remember seeing them. I don't remember seeing my son, I don't remember seeing my husband. Later, a nurse told me that they remember me being up at the hospital. They told me that my family was in my room talking to me, but I don't remember talking to them. And, I really did feel a guilt complex because I felt bad about not remembering my son being there or my husband or my family.

Towards the end of her month-long stay at the acute-care hospital, a social worker came to see her to tell her that she was going to be moved to Rehab Central, a rehabilitation hospital. Although Ida had no medical insurance, she was being admitted to Rehab Central free of charge (Ida was not charged for her acute-care hospitalization either). It was a teaching hospital attached to a university, and the social worker told Ida that the facility took in people from time to time at no charge. No doubt, the doctors thought that it would be useful for students to study Ida's recovery, and she remembers her doctor frequently coming to see her along with a group of students who would examine her and ask questions about her rehabilitation.

By the time Ida was moved to Rehab Central, one month after her stroke, she had regained normal consciousness and was able to remember her time there. She even remembers the ambulance ride from the acute-care hospital to Rehab Central, which she thought was exciting, but also difficult because she was uncomfortable lying on the gurney.

The first morning she woke up at Rehab Central, she had a horrendous headache. She was given medication for it and it went away, but she mentions this because it was something unusual for her. Her stroke was not accompanied by a headache. Once, before her stroke, her doctor had expressed surprise that she did not get headaches, considering how high her blood pressure was. She had never been given a prescription for medication, and she is not sure why but suspects that it was because she did not ask for one. In retrospect, she wishes that she had asked, particularly since, at the time that doctors expressed concern, she had medical insurance through her employer that would have allowed her to pay for the medicine.

On Ida's second day at Rehab Central, she began a gruelling rehabilitation regimen. She was surprised at how hard she was expected to work each day; she had hoped that the therapists would be gentler with her. As it was, she was kept busy with physical, speech and occupational therapy every day, from 8:00 in the morning until 5:00 in the afternoon. The only break she got was for lunch. She said that "they proceeded to work the devil out of me." Ida found all this therapy physically exhausting, and she would get back to her room ready to go to sleep.

The physical therapists were focused on helping Ida regain movement on her paralyzed right side. When she first arrived, she could not get out of bed on her own or do anything for herself. She found this strange, and would sometimes try to do something only to find that she couldn't. Also strange was that she could not feel what she was doing with her right side. For example, she said, "They had me up with some parallel bars and I was walking with the parallel bars and I was like: how am I able to walk and I can't feel my leg? So that's a weird feeling also."

Ida quickly came to appreciate how fortunate she was to be at Rehab Central where she had the opportunity for such focused therapy. She had no worries as far as her family was concerned because her mother and aunt had stepped in to care for her son, husband and uncle. Yet she was eager for the day when she could return home again, to care for her son herself. With this incentive, she pushed herself even when she didn't feel like it, working as hard as she could to regain movement and control over her right side. Having her son in mind, made her feel that she "really didn't have a choice." She was especially interested in regaining as much use of her arm and hand as possible. She doesn't think, however, that her therapist paid as much attention to helping her with this as she could have: "Well, she may have been qualified but she was also getting married, so I don't think she gave me enough attention. I think that was one of the things why, you know, I feel like I don't have much use for my hand today."

She compared her persistence in therapy with that of another woman she met at Rehab Central and befriended. Her friend seemed uninterested in working at recovery:

> We would sit in the chairs and do different exercises. And she would laugh and joke and kid and she wouldn't do hers. So when she left she was still unable to do a lot. She said to me once after we got out, "You told me I should stop playing." I said, "Yeah, it's all right to have some fun but the fun that I was having [meant] I was still doing my exercises because I wanted to get well."

Ida was discharged after a month but continued physical therapy as an out-patient for almost two years. She returned home and had home nursing care for a while. Mostly, though, her husband and son cared for her with constant help from Ida's mother and aunt. Even her disabled uncle tried to help doing things for her, which Ida thought "was sweet of him." Ida told him, though, that he shouldn't try to help her because they were both at risk of falling down. With her sardonic sense of humour, she thought it was rather funny to think about "two crips helping each other."

For the first while after she got home, therapists came to her home to work with her. There was one who worked on her arm, and one who worked on her leg. She would practise walking and learned how to do things such as walk sideways up a hill. She was especially happy with the arm therapy that she got while she was at home, and believes she made more progress with her home therapist than she had while at Rehab Central. She continued to work hard at doing her exercises. "One thing I will tell you," she said, "after they come out, then I would sleep all day the next day [laughing]! I was wore *out!*" Then, after therapists stopped coming to her home, she went back to Rehab Central three times a week for therapy.

All of this therapy, both at home and as a hospital out-patient, was at no charge to Ida, and she is extremely grateful that she was accepted as a patient. She suspects that her age may have had something to do with this. She said: "I think that my being only thirty-eight meant they probably could see a possibility of me benefiting from being there. It's an educational hospital so I guess I was a guinea pig for them."

Had she not been accepted as a patient free of charge, she would not have been able to pay for therapy herself, considering that she had no medical insurance. It's not clear, either, that she would have qualified for Medicaid, the state insurance for low-income people, because she had been employed at the time of the stroke. Even if she had qualified, she might not have received as much rehabilitative treatment. Also at no charge for Ida were the braces that she was given to help her with walking, which helped her tremendously.

Ida's marriage, meanwhile, began to deteriorate after she got home. She began to worry that she would not be able to return to being the woman she had been beforehand, and she didn't want Joseph to feel obligated to care for her. "When I had my stroke, I remember telling my husband, I said, 'Look, I understand that I've had a stroke and I don't know if I'm gonna get well or what,' and I even gave him the option of getting out of the situation," she said.

At the time, Joseph declared his continuing love for her and said that he would stay with her. Two years later, though, at the height of Ida's depression, he left. While Ida in no way blames herself for his leaving, she can nevertheless see that she was difficult to live with at the time. She was desperately unhappy and she always seemed to be angry about something. Joseph figured that she was mad at *him*, and she couldn't seem to get him to understand that it was the situation in which she found herself that she had a hard time dealing with.

It was only later that Ida found out that Joseph had actually left her for another woman. Not only that, he fathered a child with the other woman, while still living with Ida. She said:

All the time, I think what made me mad about it was that he had other reasons, so it was kind of like he used my illness against me. To justify what he did. Beforehand we had trust, and he violated the trust thing. He's made it hard for me to trust him now, because he's introduced this other woman which not only did he do the other woman thing, but he had another child. You know, out of marriage. And it seems like he just messed it up big time.

They were never divorced and continued to see each other because of their shared commitment to raising their son. Ida always made sure to take Brad to see his father on a regular basis. She took Brad to see Joseph, rather than have Joseph come to get Brad, and she felt that this gave her a freedom that she wouldn't have had if he had been coming to her place.

At the time of the interview, Joseph was trying to convince Ida that they should go back to living together again. But Ida says she's too afraid that he would do the same thing again. She doesn't see how she can ever have the kind of close emotional relationship that she used to have with him. As well, she has learned that she likes what she can do being on her own. She may not be rich, but she is financially independent. She has learned that she is very capable of taking care of herself and she has come to cherish the freedom she has because of her de facto single status:

He wants to tell me what to do. And I kind of feel resentment about that because I look at all the stuff I've accomplished without him being here. And then I kind of feel like, well, you shouldn't tell me what to do. And another thing, I can't deal with all the negativity. When he found out that I had had this apartment, instead of him saying, "Well, you done good, you found a place to stay and you're raising my son, my son is going to school," and you know. Instead of him giving me positive stuff, he's negative with it: "Well, your apartment's too small and you ain't doing this and you ain't doing that." And I guess in my mind I feel like, if you can't get your *own* life straight, don't tell me how I'm living mine. You know, I'm doing okay, I'm considering that I *am* doing okay because I'm better off than I *was*. You know, I'm not living with nobody. Not dependent on staying with somebody. I got my own place, pay the rent.

Ida went on to say that she felt taken for granted by Joseph, as though he expects her to be there for him, regardless of what he does. She also suspects that he doesn't really like who she has become without him, but that "he wants me to stay sickly." Thus, she resisted his pressure to move back in with her.

Despite the extensive physical therapy that Ida has received, her right side remains severely impaired. There is little that she can do with her right arm or hand. She used to be right-handed, but has learned to do a lot with her left hand, and if someone is around to help her with something that she can't manage, she is not necessarily averse to asking for help. Others, however, don't always recognize how extraordinarily difficult ordinary tasks can be for her. Even though strangers can look at her and see that she limps or doesn't use her right side, the disabling consequences of her stroke are not always visible to her family. Ida, moreover, believes that it's virtually impossible for them to understand what life is like for her with her impairments.

> 'Cause until you've walked and been in them shoes, there is no way you can explain this to anybody else. I know that one thing I did when I came home — my son is left-handed, but when I would call him in the kitchen to come open a can for me or twist open a jar, you know, he'd be like, "Oh Mama, you can do that." I said, "OK, you hold one hand behind your back and do it one handed." You know, and then he would be trying to do it and he'd get frustrated, you know. And I said, "You see, I'm not asking you just to be calling you in here to do stuff for me."

Over time, Ida has come to the point of being able to see the humour in a situation when she doesn't quite get something right. Sometimes, for instance, she'll put on her clothes backwards, or inside out. "I just get so tickled with myself," she said. "At first I used to get mad, but now I just laugh 'cause you have to learn to laugh at yourself."

Whereas getting dressed was once something that Ida did without much forethought — few people give a lot of thought to the mechanics of getting dressed — the activity has become something that can be quite difficult. No longer can Ida buy clothes for herself simply because she likes how they look. Now, like many of us who have one-sided weakness and difficulty co-ordinating hand-and-arm movements, she buys clothes with an eye towards practicality and whether they can be taken on and off with ease. Buttons, for instance, can be a problem, but one trick Ida has learned is to do up the buttons on a shirt before she puts it on, and then pull the buttoned-up shirt on over her head. Also difficult is putting on and taking off a bra. About this, Ida said, "The hardest thing was learning to put on a bra, oh my god! Who made bras? Oh my gosh!" Many of these techniques for one-handed dressing (and other activities) are taught to us by occupational therapists, but many of us also figure out on our own how to do things with one hand. Chris Madsen, for instance, solves the problem with bras by wearing only sports bras (which don't need to be fastened).

Ida has also stopped wearing dresses because she can't get in and out of a car in an elegant manner. Instead, she needs to open up her legs so that if she were in a dress, she would be "flashing the world." Thus, she would much rather wear a pair of pants and not have to worry about modesty or whether someone is available to help her dress. This created a problem when Ida wanted to go to church after getting out of the rehab hospital, because her church was one where it was expected that women would dress up to look their best. The first time Ida went back to church wearing pants, her aunt gave her a hard time. Ida stood her ground, pointing out that "God is looking at my heart, he's not looking at what I have on." Fortunately, people at Ida's church have come to adopt a more casual attitude towards acceptable clothing, and she is no longer singled out as being inappropriately dressed.

More troublesome for Ida than her right-sided hemiplegia is the way she so easily becomes fatigued. For the first while after her stroke, she figured that her tiredness was because she was still recovering. She thought she would soon enough return to her usual level of energy. As was the case for all the women profiled in this book, no one told Ida to expect that persistent fatigue might become a regular part of life. Thus, when she continued to become fatigued long after she thought she should be better, she would get mad at herself. She would chastise herself for not trying harder, as though she were somehow slacking off. It took her years to come to terms with this consequence of her stroke, as she began to realize that she just didn't have the stamina that she had before and there was nothing she could do about it. Now she has more respect for her limits and she makes no apology for them. Recently, a relative came to visit her and commented negatively on the state of her apartment, telling her she needed to clean it up. Ida took offence and told him to go home. Others don't seem to understand, she says, that apparently simple things can be "a monumental chore" for her to accomplish. Sometimes, things that are not essential just don't get done.

Daily life requires much more planning than it once did, but planning allows Ida to determine her priorities and pace herself accordingly. More than once, family members have been annoyed with her for her lack of spontaneity when it comes to doing things, but Ida says, "I'm not doing stuff at the last minute. No, I'm not rushing, no. I'm just not going to do it. And then people, they get mad at you for being that way." Ida cherishes whatever energy she has and is not interested in using it up to please others at her own expense.

Ida learned all this slowly. When she first got home from the rehab hospital she had a lot of help and support from her extended family, but it didn't last:

> When you come home from the hospital, everybody's there, they want to do this for you, that for you. And then all of a sudden you wake up one day and nobody's there. You know, it's like you have to call somebody to get them to do something or — and that makes you feel like — that also brings you down. Because it's just like you don't want to be a burden. I know I didn't.

At the same time, Ida disliked being treated as though she were incapable of doing anything for herself. She was used to being the one responsible for looking after others, so she was uncomfortable having other people jump up trying to anticipate her needs. If she needs help with something, she wants to be the one who asks for help. She illustrated this point with the following story about being at church dinners:

> I told the people at church, I know a lot of times when we have dinner downstairs or something they'll offer to go get it for me, and on the days that I feel good, you know, I want to get up and go stand in line, get my own plate of food. Carry it, and stuff like that. I said, "I don't mind getting my stuff for myself if I feel like it, but also I think that you all need to know that I'm not sitting out there, wanting people to do stuff for me."

Ida is sensitive about being considered lazy, and bridles when others suggest that she could do more for herself if she really wanted to. She says:

> When I really get to the point where I need you to do stuff for me, I want you to do it and not have a second thought about me trying to get you to do it just because I'm being lazy. Because they can't feel what you feeling and you know, like we were talking about, the, the *tired* thing, you know.

Ida's fluctuating energy level is key to whether she is going to be able to do something herself or need help. Yet, as also discussed in conjunction with other women's stories, fatigue is something that is felt subjectively, and we don't always know ourselves that we are fatigued until we try to do something. Then, we suddenly realize that we don't have the energy required, and we can't dredge it up as most people seem to be able to do. This can make it difficult to negotiate social relationships to our own satisfaction. Most of us are, like Ida, acutely sensitive to the charge of laziness, as we are aware of how confusing it must be for others to have us say that we are too tired to do something when there are no visible clues. One solution to the problem of fatigue is to plan everything well in advance — as Ida tries to do. This is not always possible, however, and in any case planning activities down to the last detail can become very tedious.

Another lasting impairment for Ida seems to be cognitive damage. While no doctor or therapist has ever talked to her about this, she nevertheless feels that she does not have the cognitive abilities that she once had. In particular, her attention span is not as good as it used to be. When she first got to the rehab hospital, she says, she couldn't even focus enough to watch television. Whereas she used to like reading books, she now finds it difficult to concentrate on what she's reading. Sometimes, for example, she'll see a long post on SAFE (Stroke Awareness for Everyone, an Internet site for stroke survivors) that she thinks would be interesting to read, but she usually doesn't because it's just too difficult for her to focus long enough to make sense of what she's reading.

It's not unusual that Ida was not evaluated for cognitive damage, or at least evaluated such that she was told that she was being evaluated; this is true for most of the women in this book, including myself. Indeed, all of the women profiled in this book experience cognitive difficulties, which are generally exacerbated by fatigue. Yet only three of the eleven were evaluated and got help relatively soon after their strokes. A fourth did not get an evaluation and help with her cognitive impairments until four years post-stroke, because it took that long before she realized that she had problems that someone could help her with.

For the first few months after Ida's stroke she was focused on physical recovery and she was mostly optimistic about how much she would recover. As time went on, though, and she began to realize the extent to which she would always be disabled, she started to lose her ability to remain upbeat. In retrospect, she is annoyed that no one had prepared her for this possibility when she was still in the hospital. "This is one of the things I felt that in rehab, they really didn't do. About teaching people how to deal with strokes or the different things that we go through."

She began to feel she had lost control of her life and became more and more depressed:

> I was going through a real bad depression bout. Because I really thought that nothing was — I wasn't getting any better. I couldn't see. So I just became negative towards myself, angry towards myself. Because I tend to be my own worst enemy or my harshest critic.

Had Ida been warned, while she was still in the rehab hospital, about the lengthy and uphill struggle she would face in trying to regain lost physical and cognitive abilities, and had she been told to expect debilitating fatigue if she tried to do too much, she might not have become so depressed. She might not have believed what she was being told, as many of the women in this book chose not to believe professionals who said they would "never" do this or that, or she might have believed them and become depressed then and there. It seems, though, that if she had been warned and then become depressed, then at least there would have been resources at the hospital to help her come to terms with her future. However, had she been warned and then chosen not to believe the warnings, she would at least have returned home with the knowledge in the back of her mind that the difficulties she was experiencing were to be expected. She might not have tried so valiantly to push through her difficulties, and especially her fatigue, and she might have learned a lot earlier to be kind to herself. As it was, Ida was used to being the one that others turned to for help. When she found herself unable to easily take care of herself, let alone take care of others, she not only felt that she was letting others down but she also felt that she was letting herself down. Many women take on responsibility for others, and many women become depressed when they find that they can't fulfill their own expectations about what they should be doing.

After Ida got home from the rehab hospital, she went to a specialist to get her high blood pressure under control. Through a process of trial and error, they managed to find medication that keeps it at an acceptable level, so she no longer has worries about that. But Ida believes that her depression is directly related to the blood pressure medication she takes. When she told her doctor about this, and when she said that she had thoughts about suicide, he gave her a referral to a psychiatrist, for psychiatric evaluation. She said:

> I went there and talked to a woman there, and told her how I
> felt, um, I mean, I literally think I was close to a breakdown

because I didn't know what was going on. I honestly have to tell you, yes, I was suicidal. It shocked me when I thought about that, because I was thinking to myself that I'm not the kind of person that would even consider suicide. You know, I don't believe in it, and it's part of my religion not to believe in it. But I honestly got to the point of sinking so low that I now understand why people consider suicide.

Ida saw her psychiatrist once a week. One of the first things the psychiatrist did was put her on Prozac. "Prozac is keeping me on an even keel. I feel so bad when I don't take it." She has heard of others who have been on Prozac being able to wean themselves off of it, but she doesn't see herself being able to do this. She remains convinced that it is her blood pressure medication that is primarily responsible for lowering her mood, and since she expects she will have to take that for the rest of her life, she is unable to imagine not being on Prozac or, at least, some kind of antidepressant medication.

Ida has little tolerance for irritations and red tape, such as the difficulty she's been having in getting her Supplemental Security Income cheque (disability benefits), and becomes quite indignant when things do not go as they are supposed to. She has always had a strong sense of right and wrong, and now that she is forced to fight with government bureaucracy to get what she is entitled to, she won't stand for it. At the time of the interview, for instance, her cheque was late and she was being given a run-around in order to get money to pay her rent. She went down to the office to complain:

> The woman at the window knew my situation 'cause I had talked to her before. Then they told me to go and talk to somebody in the back. They gave me to a new employee in the back. When I told this to the man, I said, "Well, the lady at the desk told me that y'all were going to cut me a cheque to pay my rent." He went through and made me answer all these questions, he fiddled around, he got up about ten or fifteen times to go ask questions, then he'd come back. He ended up telling me over all of that period of time that there was nothing he could do. And I politely told him, I said,

"Look, y'all gonna do something, my landlord is going to put me out because I can't pay my rent. This was a cheque that y'all said was going to be in the system and sent to me, it never showed up." Well, here it is another week, I still have not got my cheque. So I've got to go back down to the social security office and see what's going on with the cheque if I don't get it today. Because my rent is due tomorrow. And see that burns me up, and I even told him, I said, "Look," I said, "how can y'all do this to people that are disabled like this? And what about the people that are worse off disabled than I am?" You know.

Her patience, which she says was never her strong suit, has worn thin. She acknowledges that she has always had a "patience problem," but she now feels that she has to constantly worry about things such as medication or finances. She would much rather have things work the way they are supposed to, so that she could relax knowing that everything has been taken care of. She said:

You know, like the episode of dealing with social security and getting my money I told you about, it's a big hassle which I don't feel I should have to go through. I feel like I'm being treated wrong, maybe that's what I want to say. I want to say to them, "Look, I've got a problem that I'm dealing with that's horrendous to me, you know," but I guess I can't make society understand that and it makes me mad that they *don't* understand that and then I tend to think that, well, other people got worse problems than me. So it's like on one hand I feel bad about that, but then on the other hand I feel that I should be treated with some kind of respect. Because I feel like — the stroke to me was like, monumental. I think that if you've had a stroke, you know, you shouldn't have to *deal* with all this other stuff.

Ida is not willing to simply sit back and do nothing about the injustices she encounters:

I'm the kind of person that once I set my mind to it, I'm gonna be your headache. Like I said, if it just takes sitting here writing that man [about the disability benefits] the same letter every month, I'll do it. It don't cost me but what, thirty-seven cents? And I got a book of stamps, I will type a letter. Write it all, put it in an envelope. There it goes. So he'll get tired of me sending mail, he'll do something [laughing]. He'll be like, "Oooh, why can't y'all do something with this woman, get her to stop sending me letters?" [laughter]

I'm the advocate. You know ... you don't *do* this. Like I said, I've even thought about typing up little nasty notes to put on [cars] — and I'm gonna do that eventually, make me some little nasty notes or nasty little posters when people park in the handicapped spot. You don't have a handicapped sticker or a license plate, you know you should be ashamed to be parked here. So I figure that God has left me here, like I said, to help people that have strokes, if they need to know things about it. But also, to get on somebody's nerves and that's what I'm gonna do [laughing]!

When Ida was younger, she was afraid of disabled people and the various assistive devices they sometimes used, such as a prosthesis, braces or a wheelchair. For Ida, it was a fear of what was strange and unexplained. Disabled people were not a part of Ida's everyday world as a child, and she absorbed the culture's general fear of disability and impairment. This fear is manifested in so many ways, but one example would be the fact that many of "the bad guys" in the tradition of European fiction are identified as "bad" because of their impairments. Children, for example, learn to fear Captain Hook in the story of Peter Pan. Another example would be Shakespeare's Richard III, who was portrayed as "bad" because of his humped back. Thus, when Ida had her stroke and then found that she herself needed aids, she didn't want to accept them into her life. She credits her son with helping her to move away from that attitude and see that impairment and assistive devices are nothing to be afraid of. She began to change her mind when she was still in the rehab hospital:

And he'd take my wheelchair and go out in the halls, just rollin' all up and down the halls. And the lady that was in the room with me, her son came out and he was poppin' wheelies in her chair and he was trying to show my son how to pop wheelies. And everything I bought was supposed to be for me, my medical stuff. 'Cause I even bought this little thing that you sit on where you can turn to get out of a car, he'd sit on the floor and play, play, play twist-a-whirl with that, you know! So it kind of made me feel like, well, it's not so bad. You know, if he doesn't think it's so bad … So he helped me to see the positive side of it.

She went on to rave about the joys of freedom in her wheelchair, which she uses when she needs to get around for longer distances, such as when she wants to go shopping at the mall: "Even now when I'm in my wheelchair and I go somewhere — I love it when I get to a hill. Well, not a real steep one, but just one I know. And there's nothing in the way. I'm like, let me *go*! Let me go!"

Ida was looking for work at the time of the interview. For the first two years after her stroke, she, Joseph and their son had been living in her aunt's house rent-free. After her husband left, though, and she got her own apartment, then she began to feel that it was time to go out and get a job. It was not so much a case of needing the money, because she was getting her basic financial needs met with her disability benefits. It was more that she felt a need to get out of the house and be with other people. She said:

I didn't really look at going back to work until later. My son was growing up and plus I was home by myself and I'm just not the kind of person that would stay home by myself. I don't know; I'm just not June Cleaver [laughing]! And I guess that's where my mind is now. I want to work as long as I can.

When she first started looking for work, she found a full-time job in an office taking charge of the payroll records, and she stayed there for two years. The job got her out of the house every day, and she was able to earn some money to spend on things other than basic necessities. She ended up leaving, though, as she found it was just too much for her physically. She would come home so tired she couldn't do anything. She went back on disability, but at the same time started looking for a part-time job that she could cope with while continuing to get some benefit support. Eventually, she found a job that she thought was perfect:

The last job I had I would sit at a desk with a headphone, computer and take orders for places that sell car equipment. It was perfect, I would go in at 11:00 and stay till 3:00; perfect 'cause it was a good time. I didn't have to get up too early and could take my time; it was also very close by.

Ida did that job for about a year, but then the position was eliminated as part of a general company downsizing, so Ida went looking once again. She found a series of temporary jobs, such as one she took not long before the interview. It took too much out of her, though, and she commented: "It's amazing that we strokers can get tired at the drop of a hat, it makes me mad. I know I went on a temp job last week, and I worked from 8:30 to 4:30 and it took me two days to recoup. I definitely can't do the eight-hour thing anymore!"

Ida had no doubt that she would find work. She had, after all, spent several years being relatively successful at finding part-time and/or temporary jobs, so she knew it was just a matter of time before she found something else. Still, she felt that she was often denied work because of her impairments. She said: "It makes me so mad that they don't seem to want to give the handicapped a chance. It still mystifies me how society doesn't give the disabled a chance even though they have passed that act."

Here, Ida was referring to the 1990 *Americans with Disabilities Act* (ADA) to prohibit discrimination against people with disabilities, for which disabled people had fought long and hard. In recent years, though, ADA legislation has been significantly weakened by successful challenges in American courts, and disabled Americans are not as protected from discrimination as they were. By comparison, Canada's Charter of Rights and Freedoms (1982) explicitly protects disabled people against discrimination, and disabled people are also protected under various provincial human rights codes. These protections are stronger in Canada than in the United States, although they do not apply to all areas of life and, as with all individual rights-based protections, one must file a complaint and engage in a lengthy legal process to seek redress for discrimination. Even stronger is the *Disability Discrimination Act* in the United Kingdom, which came into effect in 1995 to make it illegal to discriminate against disabled people in employment or in the provision of goods, facilities and services (including education). This act was amended and strengthened in 2005, and the UK government now has a Disability Equality Scheme to tackle systemic discrimination and promote equality for disabled people.

Meanwhile, Ida got her own computer in 1996, a year after her stroke. Before her husband left she had little opportunity to use her computer to connect with other people who had had a stroke, which was what she longed to do. After her husband left, though, she finally had time to search for other stroke survivors. She felt a longing to connect with others, to talk to them, to ask questions, to share her own story. She had earlier investigated face-to-face groups for stroke survivors in her city, but the groups met too far away from where she lived, and because the attendees were all much older than Ida, she wasn't interested in making the special effort to go across town. She wasn't able to go out a lot, partly because it was too tiring and partly because of the expense, but she could certainly sit at her computer to make connections.

One of the first sites she found was the AOL stroke network, and she eagerly began chatting with people, but she soon found that the AOL stroke group was not very welcoming to newcomers, so she stopped visiting the site. Then she found another site where the survivors were friendlier, and she made some lasting connections with people. It was on this site that she saw the notice I had posted looking for women to tell their stories. She responded enthusiastically. She feels that she has learned a great deal from her post-stroke experiences and wants to let others know that there is light at the end of the tunnel:

> I tend to think now that God uses people as examples to let other people know that they can get through certain situations. That's the way I look at it. That I'm just here to help and try to be an example to help somebody else make it over this hump.

Ida now sees that not only is there life beyond stroke but also that a good life can be lived even with serious impairments. As with many of the other women I spoke to, her spiritual beliefs and religious community have helped her along the way. Her faith was intensified by an experience she had when she was still in intensive care immediately after her stroke. It was so powerful that she doesn't like to talk about it with everyone:

> I feel funny telling this because I don't want people to think
> I'm crazy but I do remember that, when I was in intensive care,
> I had what I want to call an out- of-body experience. Because I
> feel that God took me and showed me some things. I've told a
> couple of people maybe about this. But you know I don't think
> I need to be telling just regular people.

It's interesting that Ida had an experience comparable to Cindy Davis's experience in ICU. Both women understood them as messages from beyond: messages that told them they were not going to die because they still had work to do.

During the time that Ida was depressed with thoughts of suicide, she found it difficult to remember that God had important reasons to want her around, or if she did remember, she found it difficult to care. As she climbed out of her depression, she reconnected with her sense of self and re-established her connection with God. She was able to move forward with her life and with her newfound purpose of helping others navigate the difficult waters of surviving stroke.

*

Ida is now living on her own, as her son, now twenty-two, has embarked on a career in the U.S. Navy. He was stationed in the Gulf for six months in 2006, which had Ida on pins and needles, but he returned safe and sound to be stationed in the United States. He is engaged to be married, but Ida suspects that the wedding will not take place for some time yet. Before he joined the Navy, he was helping Ida care for her mother who had developed dementia. Ida had her mother living with her for a while, and tried valiantly to care for her, but it proved to be too difficult. So Ida was forced in 2005 to place her mother in a nursing home, which she feels guilty about, but she realizes that with her own impairments, there is no way she can adequately care for her. Meanwhile, Ida has found a part-time job that she can easily cope with, and she is pleased that she does not need to be so reliant on social assistance.

I am struck by Ida's strength of character — her willingness to push on in the face of adversity while maintaining a sense of humour. I saw this kind of strength in all of the women interviewed for this book — it shone through as they told me their stories. Perhaps all of these women are quite unusual in their fortitude, and perhaps I was fortunate to find such strong women by happenstance. Yet I am not satisfied with this explanation. I rather prefer to think that all of these women are more typical than atypical in terms of the determination with which they faced their post-stroke lives: their refusal to be beaten down, at least not for long, by circumstances beyond their control; the creativity they show in finding ways to incorporate impairment into their lives; and, what I think is especially significant, the realization of their own strengths as independent women.

Violet Carberry

LEMONS INTO LEMONADE:
THE ROLE OF SUPPORT

Violet Carberry, a woman of Anglo-Saxon descent, has survived two ruptured aneurysms. The first one was in 1986, when Violet was thirty-seven, and the second was ten years later when she was forty-seven. When I met her in May 2004, she was fifty-five. I had driven to her home in the small town of Embro, in southern Ontario. She welcomed me warmly and introduced me to her husband, who then left us alone. We went into the kitchen and after Violet made coffee, we sat comfortably at her kitchen table as she told me her story.

Even before Violet's first ruptured aneurysm, she had been through more than her share of difficulty and trauma. When she was twelve, one of her brothers was shot and killed, and when her other brother was fifteen, he died in a car accident. Violet is also a survivor of rape, which happened when she was quite young. She doesn't like talking about any of these traumatic events, and I didn't press her for details.

Violet left school after finishing Grade 10. She was married at age nineteen and when she was twenty-six, her son was born. It was not a happy marriage — her husband was unfaithful and abusive. Money was a constant worry too, and there were times when she would eat nothing but peanut-butter sandwiches because she couldn't afford anything else. Violet left her first husband and eventually remarried. It was a better marriage but it ended in tragedy — her second husband died of cancer.

In understanding how Violet coped with her strokes, it's important to recognize that her strokes were not necessarily the most traumatic events of her life. Her early experiences shaped her as much as her later strokes did, and by the time she had her first stroke, she had learned that even when bad things happen, life goes on. One thing that stands out in Violet's story is the role support has played. She has been well-supported on an emotional level by her third husband, and she also has had support from her close-knit group of friends. They have all been there for her, and Violet has never had to deal with feelings of isolation that characterize many of the other stories. She is a fortunate woman in this regard, and she knows it.

*

In 1986, about a year after she was widowed, Violet started going out with Tim. It was soon after they began dating that Violet experienced her first hemorrhagic stroke. She was thirty-seven years old. One evening, as she and Tim were about to go to bed, she suddenly felt a terrible pressure pushing on her head, "just like a vice grip." She went into convulsions and passed out for a short time. When she regained consciousness, Tim wanted to take her to the hospital but Violet didn't want to go. Because she had diarrhea and was vomiting, she just wanted to rest. Tim took her to the local hospital in the morning, and the doctor suspected neurological problems, but because Violet appeared stable and there wasn't a neurosurgeon available, the doctor told them she should come back the next day. Violet and Tim did not find this unreasonable, and went home again. When Violet returned the following day, the neurosurgeon could tell as soon as he checked her eyes that she had had a hemorrhage. Violet was given a CT scan and flown to University Hospital in London, Ontario, for surgery. She was operated on at 1:30 in the morning.

Violet spent about two weeks in hospital recovering. She thinks she had a very good surgeon. In fact, she had nothing but praise for the hospital and staff. She added that her surgeon had operated on the singer Della Reese when she had her hemorrhagic stroke. Apparently, Ms. Reese was so grateful to the hospital for her treatment there that she spent several years performing benefits for the institution. When Violet was discharged, her doctor told her that even though she was well enough to return home, she should not drink or smoke, and she should get plenty of rest. Violet's joking response was, "Well, can I have sex? If I can't, might as well stay!" Her doctor assured her sex was permitted.

Not long after she returned home, Violet found that she was unable to move her arm. About that, she says, "I had had a slight stroke, and they took me up to the doctor, but it was just a slight one, no problems and I came through that with flying colours, I had no problems, nothing."

All in all, Violet had an excellent outcome following surgery for the ruptured aneurysm, with no lasting impairments. She took a few months to get her strength back, and returned to her job at a mail-order office. The ordeal was put behind her. About a year later, she left that job and began working at the local post office. She and Tim married.

Violet was happy in her marriage to Tim, but life at home could be stressful, because Violet's teenaged son and Tim frequently argued with each other. When Violet's son moved out on his own, in 1995, things became more peaceful at home, but Violet continued to constantly worry about things. She said, "I used to worry about what people think ... somebody would say something and I'd take it the wrong way. I worried about the least little thing, anything and everything." Violet was also concerned about keeping on top of everything, to make sure tasks got done. She said she was "a go-getter" who would work outside the house all day, then come home to take care of the household. "Nothing got me down," she added.

Her job at the post office was mostly enjoyable, but it could also be extremely stressful, "because I had a boss that was hard to work for." Still, Violet stayed there for nine years, and she would have stayed longer, probably becoming postmaster herself, but, when she was forty-seven, she experienced a second ruptured aneurysm. She explained:

> I was laying down in the afternoon and the severe pain in the head again, and I said, "Tim, I think you better take me to the hospital." So he took me to town, and I told her [the doctor] that I'd already had an aneurysm, so she referred me to a neuro-surgeon. So I went in there and I had the CT scan.

The neurosurgeon examined Violet and then consulted with a colleague at Toronto Western Hospital (TWH). She wondered if Violet would be a candidate for the newly developed treatment of embolization, a procedure that could help to repair the ruptured aneurysm, but unfortunately she was not a suitable candidate. The surgeon at TWH, however, was willing to do reparative surgery. Violet was then sent home to wait for five days until the surgery could be scheduled in Toronto.

While waiting, Violet went to see her family doctor and told him that she wasn't sure she could face going through a second surgery. Her doctor told her that she had two choices: "You can either go through it and live or not go through it and die." His words certainly gave Violet "altogether a different perspective." She submitted to the surgery.

After this second operation, Violet spent three weeks at TWH. Although she thinks that her surgeon was "a fantastic doctor," what little she remembers about her experience of being at TWH was miserable. She thinks the problem was that the hospital was understaffed, as they seemed to do everything in a hurry. Regardless, the result was that Violet suffered from careless treatment. She said: "I hated to see a nurse come through the door because I knew they were going to hurt me, and that's an awful feeling, and yet I don't remember anything about TWH except that."

For example, she was catheterized five times and this caused considerable bleeding. When her husband asked a nurse about

Violet's bleeding, the nurse suggested that she was on her period. But that was not the case, and it was clear to Tim that Violet had been injured by a lack of proper attention to the catheterization procedure. As well, there was a note at the back of her bed stating that Violet had to keep her arm elevated on a pillow, but twice her husband came to visit her only to find her with her arm twisted behind her back. Violet is not sure how that happened, but she now thinks that lying in this position caused her to suffer permanent damage to her shoulder. Violet now laughs that the hospital once called Tim to ask for a donation, and Tim said, "Well, I was thinking about suing!"

The best thing about Violet's experience at TWH was her confidence in her surgeon. She remembers that prior to the operation, when she was asked to consent to it being filmed, she joked with him that he couldn't make any mistakes because it would be captured on film. In retrospect, she marvels at her forwardness and thinks that was a very outspoken thing to say. After the surgery, Violet said that he was very good at explaining to Tim everything that was happening. Having a surgeon who is willing to take the time to answer questions and explain what is going on is so important for the emotional well-being of the survivor and her family.

After three weeks at TWH, Violet was transferred by ambulance to General Hospital, a hospital closer to home. It was while at General, where she stayed about two weeks, that she really began to return to full consciousness. Her most significant memory of her stay there was that she began to suspect that she might be paralyzed, because she couldn't move her whole left side, but she was too afraid to ask because she didn't want to have her suspicions confirmed. She also remembers being tested to see if she was ready for therapy, and when doctors determined that she was, she was transferred to a nearby rehabilitation hospital.

Violet spent about two months at the rehab hospital, working to regain use of her left side. She couldn't talk very well either, but her speech gradually improved with practise. In addition to physical therapy, she underwent occupational therapy, where "we would bake cookies and learn to wash ourselves again, and I had to wash myself twice because I didn't do too good the first time [laughter]!" Violet learned how to do things with one hand: "Like how to put a bra on and turn it around and you know, basic things that made life a little bit easier." Altogether, she found these techniques very helpful.

Physical therapy was not as enjoyable. Violet said, "Learning to walk again was no problem, but the therapy on my shoulder, oh, it was painful." She progressed from using a wheelchair, which she would push herself (with great difficulty, given that she could only use her right arm), to using a cane. When she got the cane, she "used to go like a shot out of hell," and the nurse would tell her to slow down. She was so happy, though, to finally be able to walk on her own two feet.

Although she thinks she got excellent care at the rehab hospital, she was nevertheless not happy to be there. Daily routines were difficult: "You're up at six in the morning, you've got to get washed, go down to physical therapy, go to occupational therapy, and rush out and have a cigarette when you could." The lack of privacy regarding bodily functions was embarrassing. She needed to wear a diaper because she had no feeling and could not tell when she needed to use the bathroom. But when she learned that a male nurse would change it for her, she could hardly believe what she was hearing, and she joked that he should first put a paper bag over her head in order for her to be able to cope. This was just one of the more blatant examples of the indignities that hospital patients commonly face. Nurses and other hospital staff are routinely used to dealing with the human body and all that it can produce. From their perspective, there is nothing to be embarrassed about regarding the body, and their work is organized such that they are required to deal with the body in an efficient manner. From a patient's perspective, however, it can be embarrassing. Even the term diaper, which is what hospital staff generally call protective undergarments and the term Violet herself used, is infantilizing and certainly doesn't work to support self-confidence.

One of the most difficult things about being a stroke survivor in the immediate post-stroke period is that there is truly no way of knowing how someone will recover. There is such great variability in terms of whether someone will regain all of their abilities, most of them or very little, and no one can realistically predict what will happen. Some rehab professionals, therefore, prefer not to tell their patients what to expect, and it appears that this was the attitude of Violet's therapists. Yet Violet found it particularly hard to deal with not knowing what was going to happen to her. Her rehabilitation team probably could have been more sensitive to her concerns and could have taken the time to talk to her about them. She said:

> I like to be in control, step by step, and not knowing what was coming was what was scary for me, just not knowing what was going to happen next. You know, you're just like a little kid in a doctor's office: What's he going to do to me? What's he going to do to me? You know, I think just that alone, 'cause I like to be in control and know exactly what's coming and what we're going to do.

She worked hard while at the rehab hospital. Indeed, she exceeded the therapists' expectations by being able to walk after just three weeks of intense work. She began going home on weekends, but she was still not steady enough on her feet to be able to go home permanently. She also continued to be bothered by having to wear a diaper and have someone else change it for her. Her husband, though, told her that he would rather have her at home on the weekends and change her diapers than have her in the hospital, and Violet came to realize that she would just have to put up with his help if she were to enjoy weekends at home. She decided that it was preferable to be vulnerable in the company of her supportive husband than in the hospital where she was cared for by strangers.

Violet was feeling exceptionally vulnerable. She was still reeling from the shock of becoming basically helpless when she had been used to being the one who cared for others. This is a very difficult position for many women to be in — many women are proud of their care-taking abilities and it can be an important source of their identity. When they find themselves unable to fulfill their caretaking role, it can be an emotional shock. Ida King discussed this in her story, and Violet seems to have felt similarly. It's not at all that these women felt that their entire identity was tied up with being a caretaker, but it nevertheless is a real loss to find that role taken away. Both women were eager to resume their traditional roles in their families.

Recovery was a slow and frustrating process. One milestone that Violet had mixed feelings about was getting rid of her diaper so she could go to the bathroom on her own. Much as she did not like having others change her diaper for her, it nevertheless gave her a sense of security, because for a while she didn't have enough feeling to know when she needed to eliminate. When she was told she no longer needed a diaper, she said, "It's awful to say that, but I was so scared that I'd wet myself! Oh! The diaper bit, that scared me more than anything!"

Violet was also unsure about what her husband would think of her appearance and lack of ability to care for herself. Indeed, a psychiatrist came to talk to her in hospital to see if she had any questions, and Violet told her she was worried that she was so ugly her husband might not continue to love her. The psychiatrist calmed her fears by pointing out that Tim had been to see her every day while she was in hospital, and he was doing a lot for her.

Soon after Violet talked to the psychiatrist, she went home permanently. All told, she had been a hospital in-patient for almost three months. She was pleased to get away from the hospital routines and be in charge of her own schedule, to be able to sleep in and nap on the couch. She was also happy just to be in her own home again, and did not mind resuming her role as the one in charge of housework. Tim, she said, "works hard and I didn't expect him to do much. I come from the old school of the woman does the housework, I guess." Nevertheless, she said, "my husband is *so* much help." This, despite the fact that Violet did not find Tim particularly good at taking care of housework:

> He's one who gets things out and leaves them. But I managed to cope, like I got a big pool table downstairs, and when I would

wash laundry, I laid the stuff out on the pool table and folded them up and, it took me a long time, but he would vacuum the odd thing.

It bears repeating that Violet took it for granted that it was her role to be the caretaker. She was happy to have the opportunity to be creative in finding ways to fulfill that role. If Tim helped her sometimes, she was touched by his willingness to do so. Before her stroke, housework was something that Tim habitually left entirely to Violet.

For the next eighteen months, Violet continued physical therapy at the hospital three days a week. This required a half-hour drive each way, and Tim would drive her there after he finished working the midnight shift at an auto plant. She was fortunate that Tim had good health care benefits at work, so that all her therapy was paid for under the plan.

Her biggest concern, and the focus of her therapy, was her shoulder. In fact, a week after she got out of hospital, she returned as a day patient to be operated on for "frozen shoulder" (a relatively common condition — not necessarily stroke-related — that involves stiffness, pain and limited motion in the shoulder joint). Eight years later, at the time of the interview, she still was not able to lift her arm as high as her head. She has developed arthritis, as well as the beginning of osteoporosis.

Violet reached another milestone about four months after she was released from the hospital when she stopped using a cane for walking. For the first while she found it quite scary to get around without her cane to rely on. She said: "They took my cane away. That was my crutch and I was scared to go out on my own and I was oh! *scared*! Oh! But I knew I had to do it. So, you have to do what you have to do, eh!"

Indeed, the emotion she recalled most vividly about her immediate post-hospital experience was fear:

It's like you're starting over. Learning to walk again, learning to talk again, like when I first — the first weekend I got out of the hospital, I was so scared in that van, because the cars seemed to be going twice as fast as they did before. It was just scary; it's just getting back into life.

Violet was the only interviewee to so clearly comment about feeling scared as she learned to negotiate life outside the hospital, but it's a common experience. In the hospital, we may not like the impersonality that often occurs, or we may not like the lack of control we have over what and when something happens, but we at least can feel secure about being in a safe environment where no one is judging us about how we look and no one expects us to be able to walk or talk clearly. All that changes when we leave the hospital and are confronted with the fact that the world goes on without stopping to take our needs into consideration. Typically, we become aware of just how physically unprepared we are to negotiate the fast-paced world.

Violet credited her husband with helping her get through the recovery and the rehabilitation process. She said, "He was fantastic, oh! He *really* helped me get through it." Tim would push her to get out of the house when she would have rather stayed at home. Especially at first, Violet was self-conscious about how she looked. She said, "I wouldn't go out, I didn't want to go and let people see me with a cane and with my arm funny. I didn't want people to see me like that." She thought she "looked a mess." But Tim would not let her stay home all the time. "He'd say, 'No, c'mon, we're going out for brunch' or 'C'mon we've got to go get groceries.' He did help so *much* in the mental part of it." Violet always came away from these outings feeling better about herself, because she had a good time being out with others.

After eighteen months, her physiotherapist felt she had reached a point where she would not be able to get any better, so she recommended that Violet stop therapy. Especially since driving to the city for therapy was not always easy, Violet decided to stop going. For that year and a half, though, she gave it all that she could. It was, she said, a long and drawn out process, but in the end it was definitely worth it. She didn't see that she had a choice about it, she was so determined to get better. So she pushed herself. Her son told her, "Mom, you're a fighter," and Violet's bowling league gave her a plaque for determination. She was so touched that she cried.

Violet continues on her own to do exercises to keep her arm as functional as possible, though she no longer organizes her life around recovery. To a large extent, she is resigned to her impairments. Regarding the use of her left side, Violet is grateful that she was right-handed before the stroke, because it is now very difficult for her to use her left hand for anything. She continues to have significant balance and co-ordination difficulties because of her left-sided weakness. Even now, she said, she tends to be cautious about doing things that require balance. For example, a few weeks before the interview, she got up on a little step-ladder to clean a window and fell. Luckily she wasn't seriously injured.

One thing she does that she thinks helps her to have better balance is walk. Although Violet was the only one to mention the therapeutic effects of walking, the more one walks, the easier it becomes. She and her husband have a trailer at a park not far from where she lives, and Violet spends a lot of time there during the summer. At the park she has a next-door neighbour she likes to go walking with twice a day. On average, Violet says, she walks about three miles a day with her friend. She finds that the walking has helped considerably. She has even managed to improve her ability to dance since she began her regular walks.

Violet has her cane, a walker and a commode sitting in her basement. Though she continues to be unsteady on her feet when she first gets up in the morning, or if she needs to get up in the middle of the night, she is determined not to rely on any aids, and she has told the local Legion that if anyone should need them, she would be happy to donate them.

From Violet's perspective, it is better to push herself as much as she can, even further than what feels comfortable. Her fear is that if she returns to depending on mobility aids, she might lose her ability to get around without them. In this regard, Violet is judging herself against the ableist standard that dictates it is always preferable to get around without any aids (yet this is something of a double standard given that many people rely on automobiles or even bicycles to get around).

Violet tires easily since her second hemorrhage. She said, "If I vacuum, say upstairs, I got to rest for a while. Or if I vacuum the living room and the kitchen, I got to rest for a while, and before I used to go right through the house and now I know I can't."

She also has short-term memory loss, though she did not even realize this until after she was released from hospital and started getting back into life at home. Once, shortly after she got home, she put a pot of soup on the stove but forgot to shut the stove off. She needs to write everything down, and is easily confused by having two or three things to do. She has never sought help about this, as she doesn't think there is anything that can be done. She has "just learned to live with it."

Violet is right that there is nothing than can be done to fix her memory problems. There are strategies that can be learned to compensate for cognitive difficulties, such as writing things down and leaving notes for herself in places where she'll be likely to see them, but Violet has managed to learn these strategies on her own. Unlike Cindy Davis, who was greatly troubled by her cognitive difficulties and felt a need to seek professional help, Violet considers her difficulties as more of a minor annoyance.

Due to her short-term memory loss and her inability to use her left side, Violet has been unable to return to work. She tried to return to work at the post office, but found that there was nothing she could do. She says, "They tried me out on different things but I couldn't even hold the mail in my left hand to put it in the mailboxes and they said no, that you're better to put your resignation in." So Violet sent in her resignation, and she hasn't tried to return to work since then. She received $1,200 in severance pay but she was not able to get a pension from the post office, because she had only worked there for nine years instead of the requisite ten.

At first, Violet was distressed that she could not return to work. "I miss working with the people, *that* bothered me." But, she said, "I just made up my mind, there's nothing you can do about it, so forget about it. It wasn't meant to be."

She also missed earning her own income. She had worked all her life and was used to having her own money to do with as she pleased. Although she was getting a small widow's pension each month, it was not enough to take care of all her needs. When she was unable to return to work, therefore, she found herself in the position of having to ask her husband for money. She said she felt guilty about asking, even though Tim told her not to. "But I did," she said, "you know, every time I wanted to get my hair done, can I borrow ten bucks or can I have twenty bucks for my books? And, I hated it."

Eventually, she applied for and managed to get a disability pension from the government. The process of getting the pension, though, was very difficult. When she first applied she was refused, so she got a lawyer. She learned that to fight for her case she would have to go to an occupational therapist for an assessment. It would cost $1,200 and would involve two full days of assessment. Her difficulties with getting certified as disabled for the purpose of getting her disability pension are typical — many Canadians find that it can be a lengthy and expensive ordeal. When Violet learned what she had to do to fight her case, she was ready to give up because she didn't have that much money, but her husband wanted her to persist. If for no other reason, he told her, she should fight for the principle of the matter. Her case went before a tribunal board, and almost two years later, she managed to get her pension. She said that her doctor was very angry that Violet had to fight so hard, considering all the impairments she had been left with.

Although she only gets a little more than $400 a month, she is happy to now have her own income:

> That's all I wanted, I just wanted enough that I didn't have to go to Tim and ask every time I wanted a dollar to get my hair done or I wanted to buy a book or something. [Once I was given the money], I didn't have to go to him and ask ... four hundred's fine with me, just a little bit of spending money of my own, and that gave me a lift.

As Violet says, financial independence is important for her on an emotional level. Not since she was a child had she been in the position of having to depend on someone else for money. She had always paid her own way, and she was used to having this level of control over her life. In this respect, she was much like Ida

King who had also been used to earning her own income since she was young. In Violet's case, her $400 a month did not give her complete financial independence from her husband, but it was enough for her to regain a small measure of control over how she spent her money, so that she was not totally dependent on his goodwill.

Friends have also been very important for Violet as she rebuilds her post-stroke life. They are all aware of her impairments, and she feels she can count on them to look out for her. She has what she calls her winter friends and summer friends. Her winter friends are from her bowling league, and she has known them for almost twenty-five years. Violet and Tim often go out with them. Recently, they've done things such as go to the Shakespeare Festival at Stratford (about this, she laughs, "We're getting so couth now!"), and they've been to a local motel that puts on a murder mystery. Violet's summer friends are comprised of about ten couples with whom she spends time when she goes out to her trailer. They all do things together such as play bocce ball. Of her summer friends, she said, "It's just like a big happy family." Violet will sometimes go out to the park on her own because Tim is working and can't get away, and she feels that she is in very good hands there. She says the people there would take care of her in a minute if she needed help. "Oh, they're great out there, a great bunch."

At first when Violet came home from the hospital, she didn't like asking for help because she thought she should be pushing herself to do things on her own. But she came to accept that there were things she could no longer do, and now she is not shy about asking for help when she needs it. She said, "I do a lot of stuff on my own but if I can't do it I'll ask for help." Her attitude is in keeping with her attitude towards helping others in general. She strongly believes that people need to try helping themselves before they ask for help from others.

Despite Violet's residual impairments and her constant awareness of not being able to use her arm as she would like, she does not identify as a disabled person. To a large extent, she says, this is because she is proud, and to a lesser extent, disability represents helplessness to her. Yet she also says that disability is not an issue she has ever thought about, so she can't say with any certainty what she thinks about the subject.

Rather than focusing on what she can no longer do, Violet focuses on what she still can do. There was never a time, she said, when she felt sorry for herself over what had happened to her. She said, "I didn't think of it that way. I thought of it that I'm lucky to be alive and I thank the good Lord that I've done as well as I have." Indeed, considering that she has lived through two ruptured aneurysms, Violet thinks that she has done "fantastic."

Nor does she worry about "petty things" any longer, and she now takes time to enjoy "little things, like the birds and the butterflies." When she goes out to the trailer park, she loves to sit and watch the squirrels, which is something she could do for hours. She has always been an animal lover, but before she became disabled, she was always too busy to sit and enjoy them. Now, she makes a point of making sure that she takes time to rest every day. Violet also feels she is a happier person than before her stroke. She said, "I think before, there was so much stress and like I'd worry and stew and *now* I just don't let stuff bother me. I live for today and live it to the fullest."

More than anything, she is thankful for what she has: "I thank the good Lord for the little good things — I got my health, I can pay my bills, and I got food on the table and a nice trailer. 'Cause I do live a good life. It couldn't be any better."

At the same time that Violet recognizes the changes in her life, she doesn't think that her core self has changed as a result of her stroke experiences. Certainly she has been forced to reorganize how she does things, but she doesn't feel that she is any different from who she was, and her basic attitudes towards other people have not changed. What *has* changed is that she has become aware of how tenuous life can be: that anyone can be "here today, gone tomorrow." She came to this awareness gradually, she said. At first, she did not want to think about how close to death she had come. Now, however, she thinks about how fortunate she was to survive when she hears of so many others who die almost immediately.

Instead, she considers herself very lucky to be alive. Her attitude is: "You get thrown a lemon, you make lemonade with it!"

*

By the time of Violet's stroke, she was already a survivor of some extremely traumatic experiences. Consequently, she had already developed skills for coping with life's adversities, and in a sense, she was much better prepared than many other women for dealing with the trauma of stroke and permanent impairment. She is creative in her ability to adapt to her circumstances and make the best of her situation. Precisely because she doesn't take it for granted that she is entitled to anything (life has taught her that), she is grateful for what she does have. Moreover, what she has "in spades" is a strong support network made up of her husband, her son and her friends. Perhaps if more stroke survivors were able to count on such extensive support from people who accept them as they are, there would be fewer reports of post-stroke depression and a lot more reports of women turning lemons into lemonade.

Jean Barton

THE JOY OF SINGING:

REHABILITATION

Jean Barton's hemorrhagic stroke occurred shortly before her fiftieth birthday. Jean, who is Jewish, lives in Manchester, England, and was fifty-six when we met for our interview at her home in 2002. She greeted me warmly when I arrived at her doorstep and ushered me into her kitchen with its large windows affording a view of her back garden. She apologized for the state of the garden, saying she had not been able to do much with it lately. As it was December, however, I commented that from my Canadian perspective, I was amazed to realize that anyone did anything with an outside garden at that time of year. We continued to chat and get to know each other, and she told me about her experiences.

So many of the themes that are in other stories also appear in Jean's: negotiating work and career, invisible impairment and feeling like the "other," and the significance of support. All of these experiences, however, are conditioned by Jean's overarching experience of not having had rehabilitation offered to her at an early stage.

*

In April 1996, forty-nine-year-old Jean Barton had been happily married to Ed for twenty years. It was a good marriage, although neither Jean's nor Ed's family entirely approved of it. Jean's family disapproved because Ed was not Jewish and was from a lower social class. Ed's family, meanwhile, disapproved because Jean was Jewish and from a higher social class. As Jean says, religion was the official reason given for why the families disapproved, but in her opinion, "My parents were being snobs and his mother was an anti-snob!"

When they married, Jean and Ed had hopes for their own children, but they were unable to conceive a child. Nevertheless, they built a happy life for themselves. They had been quite involved in the lives of their nieces when they were young, as well as the children of their best friends, and so they did not feel that they had missed out completely on the experience of raising children. Once the children were grown, though, they went off to lead lives of their own and did not maintain frequent contact, which saddens Jean.

Jean was working as a hospital technician but she had come to hate the job. The work had become automated and she felt like "an underfunded robot." She missed the hands-on work and was thinking about a major career change. Her dissatisfaction was intensified after she was diagnosed with breast cancer in 1990 and had to have a double mastectomy. After surviving that life-threatening crisis, she was less interested in putting up with a job that gave her no pleasure. She started thinking about what else she would like to do. Still, she didn't want to jump into something new until she had reached the important five-year mark of living cancer-free. Finally, in October 1995, she was able to breathe a sigh of relief over her medical exam — it showed no sign that her cancer might return. She was thrilled to have another chance at life and feels that her mastectomy was "a small price to pay."

She enrolled in a holistic massage-therapy course with the goal of setting up her own practice. The people on whom she worked during her training told her that she was good, and that they'd be interested in going back to her. Jean was encouraged by these comments and said, "It was going really well. I mean, it was just absolutely right for me." Her husband Ed was supportive of her plans. They had discussed the financial consequences such a move would probably bring and decided that they could cope with whatever happened as she established herself in a new career. By April 1996, she had only three more months to go before graduating with her massage-therapy diploma. She could hardly wait for the day when she could hand in her resignation from her job at the hospital. The stress of the job had her losing weight, getting indigestion and sleeping poorly. She was, she said, "like a coiled spring," and recalls thinking, "If I don't get out of this place, I'll go mad!" Things finally seemed to be coming together for Jean.

Yet, in recent years, Jean had been having periods of feeling unwell. Once every few weeks, she would get pain on the right side of her face. She went to her doctor about it and was diagnosed with, as she says, "something called atypical facial pain." Around January, she was referred to a neurologist who ordered a CT scan for her, but "nothing showed up." Apparently, it was just something she had to suffer through. Thus, when she was enjoying herself at home one Saturday afternoon and she started having a right-sided headache, she wasn't terribly alarmed:

And this was similar but much worse, and my thought was, oh, it's the same again but this is worse than usual. And I came downstairs, popped my head round the door, "Ed, I've got a bloody awful headache, I'm going to take some Aspirins and go to bed." I lay down on the bed, went to sleep, and woke up a week later.

Jean had had a hemorrhagic stroke. She only knows what Ed has told her about how she got to the hospital and was diagnosed:

Apparently he tried to wake me up [from my nap]. He waited an hour or so because he knew that when I had these face pains, I used to fall asleep with Aspirins. And then after two hours, he thought, right, she should be coming round, and I didn't. He tried to wake me up ... This was about nine or ten at night, and he rang the doctor who said, "Headache, go to your nearby pharmacy and I'll prescribe something over the phone," just like that. They gave him some — I think it was codeine, and he came back and thought right, that's all very well as she's unconscious, what use is that! He rang again, a doctor turned up, another one. The second one made a house call, did a few [tests], and he said vaguely, "I suppose you'd better go to hospital." Didn't phone through or anything, just gave Ed a form, I believe. When we got there, apparently I was in A and E [Accident and Emergency, the UK equivalent of the North American ER] for quite some time, I think it was the next morning when somebody had a look and did a scan and discovered I'd had a hemorrhage on the right temporal lobe.

I gather I was sort of appearing to sort of move and look around, but I wasn't actually conscious 'cause I have no knowledge of it. And they decided to send me to the National Hospital. And when I got there sometime on the Sunday, I believe they were going to wait a bit and see if it would retract, but apparently on the Monday night I started to nosedive a bit. Apparently they called the surgical team out in the middle of the night and operated and found a rather large clot.

Jean spent the next week at NH, but was mostly unconscious while there. At one point, she says, she woke up to find herself someplace where "it was all white." She had no idea where she was. Then she quickly drifted back into unconsciousness. Sometime later she woke up again, this time feeling itchy. She tried to get up:

> I realized I was lying on something. I thought, "Ooh, I've got to do something about this," and I sort of walked two steps. Something caught my feet, apparently it was the catheter and I just remember going flat on my face, lying on this floor thinking, "Now what?" And then that was it, I was out again.

She next came to consciousness as she was being prepared to be moved back to Berwick, her local hospital:

> Then I woke up again and I appeared to be in a ward. And a nurse came along and said, "Oh, we're taking you to Berwick." I thought it was a bit strange at the time, I thought, "Oh yes,

well, what's going on?" And she said, "Drink this," she put my dressing gown on, next thing I knew I was being wheeled out, put into an ambulance. The driver very kindly informed me what had happened, he said, "You've had a blood clot on the brain. And you're going to Berwick." And I thought, well, somebody's told me, that's nice.

Jean recalls being "somewhat surprised" at the news of her stroke, but said:

I didn't flip, I didn't think, "Oh my god!" I just thought, "Oh!" So it did come as a surprise, but I didn't panic at that stage, it was just, "Oh, that's what I'm doing here." I'm surprised at how calm I was at that particular point.

She spent the next three weeks recovering at Berwick. She was still unconscious more than she was conscious, but she does recall a little about her time there. There were two things in particular that were going on that worked to make her time at Berwick memorable in an unwelcome way. First, because she was sleeping most of the time, she ate very little. Orderlies would bring her meals and leave them, but no one thought to wake her up. Someone would then return some time later to remove her tray, but more often than not Jean was still sleeping, so she missed the meal. At one point, she recalls, "The nurse got a bit shirty with me," demanding to know why Jean wasn't eating, as though she were refusing to eat on purpose. Jean recalls wondering why no one would come to wake her up. In any case, it was because she wasn't eating that she was sent home after about three weeks.

The second unpleasant thing was that Jean suffered a return of eczema which she hadn't had for many years. She was allergic to chromium and nickel, and this was what the bedrails were coated with. When Jean was first admitted, Ed had indicated her allergies on the intake form. But every time he came to visit Jean he had to ask the nurses anew to cover the bedrails so that she wouldn't touch them with her bare skin. Jean said: "I was itching from head to foot. I had head-to-foot eczema. Which is not what you want when you [are recovering from a stroke]."

Fortunately, a dermatologist came to see her and brought her some cream that took care of the itching. But a nurse came and "the nurse immediately decided I was using it too much and put it away. We had to get it back from her." Then Jean started sweating because she was in a bed covered with plastic. Ed tried to get her a bed that wasn't covered in plastic, but that only happened after "a great number of threats with god knows what." About all of her uncomfortable experiences in the hospital, Jean said that "nobody noticed."

Jean went on to comment that her hospital experience was not unusual. She is reluctant to criticize the nursing staff for her poor experiences, saying, "It's not their fault. They've got so many exams to do and they don't have enough time." Yet she also points out: "It doesn't need money to just make a note and stick it on a bed: 'Leave this covered over.' Or, 'Remember to wake her up,' or something. How much does it cost? So I survived in spite of them."

When she left the hospital to finish her recovery at home, Jean was not in good shape. She was very weak because she hadn't been eating, and she could barely stand or walk. Ed took two weeks off to stay home and help her, but then he had to go back to work. Jean said:

> When I'd been home from the hospital for a few weeks, my brother said he was concerned. When Ed got home from work, he had to help me have a shower, I was so wobbly, no *way* would I do it on my own then. My brother was saying, "Maybe somebody could come and give you a hand with something," and he rang the hospital. [The person I spoke to said], "Oh, we'll send a social worker." It took her a half an hour for her to tell me I wasn't eligible for anything and that was it. 'Cause I just said, "If somebody could come in now and again just to give Ed a break, just to give me a hand with the shower or something." I wasn't old enough initially — if you were over fifty-six, you qualify for this, that and the other, but there was nothing doing. So I got to the stage, do it yourself or do without.

Jean's friends were wonderfully supportive and helpful while she recovered at home. As she says, "You soon find when something goes wrong who your true friends are. And they are." Her birth family was less supportive. Her mother — who died a year before Jean's interview — had never been willing to accept that Jean had been left with limitations and didn't seem to understand why Jean wouldn't make a three-hour trip to visit her. Jean was unable to travel very far — since the stroke, moving vehicles made her feel "very peculiar." Her mother did come to see Jean a few times, but Jean did not have a good relationship with her and found her visits stressful. Others in her family would try to tell her what to do:

> Some of my family have been known to say, "You should have been doing this, why aren't you doing that?" They have no idea. My brother used to lecture me, he was trying to tell me that I ought to have a personal trainer. I wasn't even sure what [that was]. I mean, some of my family, their idea of helping was telling my husband what he should have done, which wasn't a whole lot of good.

Meanwhile, upon release from the hospital, Jean was referred back to the same neurologist she had seen several months earlier about her facial pain. One of the first things he did was check her blood levels to see if he could find why Jean was still feeling dopey four weeks after her hemorrhage and three weeks after her surgery. He found that the anticonvulsant medication she was taking was the problem; she was taking far too much and there was a toxic amount of the drug in her blood. After they had sorted out which drugs Jean should be taking and how much, he sent her to a neuropsychologist for cognitive testing.

On Jean's first visit, the neuropsychologist commented, "I'm surprised they didn't send you upstairs to the twelfth floor, where there's the regional rehab unit." This took Jean by surprise; she hadn't known there was one there. She was also dismayed to realize that no one had thought to mention stroke rehabilitation to her before. By the time she heard about the rehab unit, she was several months post-stroke, and she had already "learned to cope with things as best one does." Nevertheless, she looked into getting accepted as a patient. In December, eight months after her stroke, she went in for two weeks.

In the rehab unit, Jean worked on her balance and co-ordination. Unlike so many others, she had never been paralyzed by her stroke. Perhaps it was because she had never been paralyzed that she was not referred for physiotherapy after discharge from the hospital. But both sides of her body had become unco-ordinated, and she lost her balance extremely easily. She couldn't stand for very long before she would start "swaying like a tree in the breeze." She describes what they did at the rehab unit:

The first thing they did, the physio got me to the gym and sort of got me fit again because for eight months I was so worried, I was frightened to go out. I mean, I could walk round the house holding on to things and gradually sort of crawl around the garden but I was frightened to go out on my own because I was so wobbly. So they got me on an exercise bike and a few weights and got me fit again. Then they took me out on the bus, made sure, you know, I should get used to going on a bus and things like that which was a start, you know.

And the other thing which she did was very much a long shot. There's a series of exercises designed for people who have balance problems with the inner-ear problem. And she said that the reason for your balance is different, but the idea is it re-educates your brain. And it starts off with — you score yourself — you start off with simple eye movements and head movements and you work down to body movements. Now, I tried and they are called dizziness-inducing exercises. I would call them nausea-inducing [laugh]! Thank god I never threw up, but I didn't feel too brilliant. I stuck to it for three months. Now, okay, it didn't solve the problem. But it *taught* me which movements were making me lose my balance. Before I'd fall over or get very dizzy and think, why did that happen? What did I do? Then I discovered with these exercises that, for example, upper-body-twisting movements. So if I turned suddenly to look at something, that was doing it. So at least I knew what to avoid which made life a *whole* lot easier even if it didn't solve the problem.

Jean also saw an occupational therapist at the rehab unit, but did not find these sessions quite as helpful. She says, "Her main function I think, to be honest, was to describe in the report what I couldn't do, which got me my retirement." When she was first admitted there, she was encouraged to think that she was finally going to get some help with her difficulties. "Just the fact somebody was doing something" was important to her. Also, "to actually get to a place where a lot of people had had strokes and talk to other people helped as well." Still, she was dismayed to see that the other patients were in much worse shape than she was. About this, she said:

> I ended up with a tremendous guilt complex. I know this sounds crazy, but there were a lot of people in wheelchairs, some of whom could walk a few steps, some of whom couldn't. My roommate couldn't speak. She was a great one for getting me doing things: "*Uh! Uh!*" She was good at the "uh"-and-point. But I thought — I felt a bit of a fraud. I thought, there are all these people who can't talk, who can't walk, and all right, I've got a shaky hand or a balance problem, I have no right to complain. Except there was one moment towards the end, I just went over to pick something up and went flat on my face, and someone said, "Good god, you lose your balance that easy?" And maybe after, I didn't feel quite so — well I didn't feel guilty for being there, so guilty for complaining if you like.

Jean's experience here speaks to one of the more troubling aspects of having invisible impairments. Given a dominant culture in which we learn to focus on and take seriously that which is visible, and discount that which is invisible, many of us with unseen impairments learn to internalize the view that the difficulties we experience aren't as serious as someone else's more visible problems. No one has studied whether women are more likely than men to feel guilty for using resources when impairment is not immediately obvious, but it would stand to reason that this might generally be the case. Women learn in so many ways that they are judged by their appearance; therefore, they not only tend to be sensitive to the gaze of others they also internalize that gaze and police themselves before anyone can judge them negatively. Thus, it's not surprising that Jean felt a little fraudulent getting help at the rehab unit. She looked around and saw visible signs of people in much worse shape than she was. She had a hard time making herself believe that her own impairments needed to be taken as seriously as those of others. A similar issue arose for Katherine Price, she felt she was doing something wrong by using her disabled parking placard. Even though Katherine had difficulty walking, she nevertheless felt that because she didn't use a wheelchair, she wasn't as entitled to a disabled parking space as someone who couldn't walk at all. In Jean's case, one wonders as well whether it was the invisibility of her impairments that prevented her doctor at Berwick Hospital from referring her for rehabilitation. Perhaps Jean was not the only one inclined to discount the seriousness of what was not immediately obvious.

All in all, Jean feels that she benefited from her brief stay at the rehab unit. She wishes, though, that she had been able to go to rehab much earlier in her recovery process: "If I'd gotten there right away they might have been able to do more." One of the best things about being there was her chance encounter with a music therapist:

> One day, a lady brought my roommate in and introduced herself and she said, "I'm a music therapist." Now, I hadn't said a word to them, because *how* could it be that important. I sang in a choir for a few years before the stroke. Straight after the stroke, surprise, surprise, I didn't feel like singing. But one day when I was feeling a bit better, I was washing up and tried to sing and it had gone completely. Nothing. And at the time, you think, well, if there's people who can't walk, talk, even for the fact I couldn't hold things straight, it's hardly that important. It was devastating, but I didn't say anything to anybody because I thought, "How can it be even important?" And when I met her, I said, "Oh god, I wonder if you could help."

Again, we see Jean downplaying the seriousness of something that was not visible. She had already decided, in her own mind, that her inability to sing was not a significant impairment (Jean did not explain *why* or exactly *how* she couldn't sing). From another perspective, however, it was of enormous emotional significance.

Her loss of that ability was devastating. Jean continued:

> And she said, "Come next door." [There was a piano in the next room.] She'd never heard about this, and she just sort of played odd notes and said, "I'd like to work with you because I've never *seen* this before. I think it's neurological." It wasn't my hearing. She played a note, if I heard it long enough I could actually hum that note.

Meanwhile, Jean had been working with the neuropsychologist to improve her cognitive abilities. The stroke had seriously damaged her short-term memory. She said:

> At the beginning I was quite sure I was talking complete sense. I discovered afterwards, that because of my short-term memory problem, I would say things twenty times over. I wasn't aware of this. I was aware that sometimes I'd say something and everybody'd start laughing. Sometimes I'd realize my mispronunciations were wonderful. Our family favourite: that tree over there is a eucalyptus. In those days, it was a eucalipstick [laughing]. So I mean, some of them I was aware of. Sometimes people had to explain. And the first time I tried to write a very simple letter, just a letter of sympathy to someone, when I looked at what I'd written, I couldn't *believe* it. It was complete rubbish, and I was told I was talking with everything the wrong way round [laughing]. I was able to speak and I wasn't hunting for a word. It was just what came out was what Ed called my reinvention of English grammar [laughing].

Particularly troublesome when she first got home from hospital was remembering whether she'd taken her medication. This was why, when she saw the neurologist, it was discovered that she was taking too much. Jean said:

> My solution was to have my teddy bear sitting on the bed with a little card saying, "Take your tablets." And then I used to have a calendar and cross off the date when I'd taken it, which I still do. And, this sounds crazy, in the kitchen — I was able to cook after a while — if I had to put six spoonfuls in something, in the early days, I had to make six marks and cross them off 'cause I'd forget, something would make a noise and I'd forget. So [by the time I saw the neuropsychologist], that sort of thing I'd already worked out.

It's astounding that Jean was not evaluated for cognitive or physical rehabilitation before discharge from hospital. In the case of memory in particular, it actually meant that Jean was in danger of either under- or overmedicating herself. As is the case for other women in this book, it would have been helpful for her to have received help much sooner than she did.

Six years later, she still has trouble remembering things. "I spend a lot of time writing things down," she said. "Thank god for Post-It notes! Otherwise I'll forget things that easily. If I don't write something immediately down or put it on a calendar, it's gone. Or I get things the wrong way around."

In the early months of her recovery, her difficulty with remembering things affected her ability to read. She is now better at remembering what she's read, but she still finds reading difficult because of the great effort required to focus or concentrate on anything. She said:

> At the very beginning, if I read a sentence, I'd get to the end and I'd forget the beginning. So to read a paragraph would take a day. Now I can actually cope with the sentences and things, but I find if I read more than for a few minutes my eyes get heavy and I get dizzy, so nowadays it takes me about the whole month to read my gardening magazine. So I haven't managed to read through a book and I used to be a great book-worm. I could never understand why this happened, but apparently somebody said it's that when you're reading, your eyes are making movements all the time. As the psychologist at the rehab explained it, [typically, our] brain gets input from all these senses all the time and filters out what it doesn't need. Mine doesn't. If I'm in a room with a ticking clock, I can hear the tick all the time. Sometimes I can hear the blood in my ears and apparently this is part of it: if you're reading, your eyes moving, you're conscious of it. See, if I want to even just read something very small — I mean, we're all right in here [in the kitchen] because had we been in there with the traffic, I'd have been losing track all the time. So I miss reading and that sort of thing.

Her problems with focusing or concentrating on things extend into many areas of life. For instance, if she's in a group situation with a lot of people talking at once, she's not able to follow what's being said: "If you're talking one to one, it's okay, but if there's a lot of people talking at once, I can't sort it out." The slightest noise distracts her, and for this reason she doesn't want to drive a car.

Jean is grateful for all the various therapists who have seen her and tried to help her, but no one has helped her quite as much as the music therapist she still sees, five years later. She said:

> I mean, I think that's why my memory is coming back and things. It helped my co-ordination. The first year I was just sitting there, poking an odd note, listening. It was helping my listening and helping my co-ordination, it was a year before she tried anything with the voice. I managed to sing after four years — that came back. I was the sort of person, I'd be singing whatever I was doing, gardening, washing, I was always sing-ing, all sort of jobs.
>
> My memory increased, for both notes and numbers and words, and at the time, I had a feeling the music was making things getting better rather than the other way around. There was an article in the *Telegraph* not so long ago, where they ac-tually believe this is the case. And they reckon it's linked to all sorts of things, so now it's thought that maybe I'm right.

Jean is just so absolutely delighted to have been in the right place at the right time to meet the music therapist. It's unlikely that anyone would have thought to refer her to a music therapist. Music therapy is not something that is routinely offered to stroke survivors, although there is growing evidence that it can be very helpful for improving not only cognitive abilities but also balance and co-ordination — all of the things with which Jean was having difficulties. When she found that music therapy was helping her not only to sing but also to improve her co-ordination, she felt she had been handed an unexpected bonus, and she is extremely thankful to have chanced upon this underappreciated therapy.

She is a creative woman, and so her post-stroke lack of co-ordination has been a blow that has forced her to give up some cherished hobbies, such as making enamelled jewellery. Yet she chooses to focus on what she *can* still do. She said:

> I can't sing in the choir again, I can only do a bit of the tune, but at least to discover I am still creating something — it's not music you would recognize but it's still some form of music. And the fact is that I still go once a week; it takes all of my benefit just about, but it's worth every penny.

What Jean misses more than anything, though, is an ability to travel. It's not only car travel that makes her feel ill, but any kind of public transit:

> I haven't been out of the city for six years 'cause barring a little tootle on the train it's more than I can cope with. I can just about manage short hops, but when I go to music therapy and I get off most people think I'm drunk, because that particular bit sways or bounces and I do feel nauseous. Thank god I never throw up. It's just that I feel pretty "ugh." And I get so dizzy, sometimes I get out the other end and it's hanging on to things and lurching from one thing to another. I get some very strange looks! And the one time I tried a longer journey — unfortunately a friend of ours died, we went to the funeral — I was in the car for about an hour and a bit. I was not much use to anybody at the other end.

As for buses and trains, she explained:

> If it's a train [I have to sit]. I did try once standing up holding on to something. I was *so* wobbly. I thought, never again. I'll just wait for another train. I mean, occasionally I do ask for a seat. I remember once I asked somebody, I said, "May I sit down, I'm disabled." And she sort of looked down and sort of shrugged, but she actually got up. Usually I don't travel in the busy times. The main problem on the bus for a lot of people is the second the last person has paid, they start off with a jerk and it can be pretty difficult.

She can't ride escalators, either, without feeling very dizzy and ill and often falling as she tries to get off at the top.

Jean's problems don't end with getting off or out of a moving vehicle, walking is a daily challenge. She doesn't like to carry a cane, even though it can be useful to help her balance and it also signals to others that she has trouble walking. She finds, however, that it gets in the way more than it is helpful. She says she has "learned to lean on walls" — something she will do even though she will "get the funny looks." She is less concerned about "funny looks," though, than she is about her own sense of safety. She recounts a sad story about one time when she was pushed and lost her balance:

> The one very nasty moment I did have — there [was] a stadium up the road. And there was one time I was coming home and there were so many fans I couldn't believe. They were screaming, so first of all there was the noise. And I was walking, thank god, I was walking on the inside, and some fan went marching past, I was in his way. He didn't say anything, he just [pushed me]. And I went whoosh, straight over, up — well, I just smashed into the wall and I was just hanging on for dear life and I couldn't go anywhere. I was shaking, and all these people, they walked past, either ignored me or laughed at me. And I think that was a matter of pride, I was just crying 'cause I didn't know what I was going to do. And not a single person said, "Are you all right? What's the problem?" In the end I thought, "Sod it, I can cope," and I got up and staggered home feeling very sorry for myself. That zapped my confidence. For several weekends when there were matches, I wouldn't go to exercise.

Her difficulties are compounded by the fact that there are no visible signs to clearly indicate to anyone that she has impairments:

> A lot of well-meaning people say to me, "You don't look as if you've had a stroke." Which is true, because I don't have one-sided impairment and, dare I say, I never stopped talking. As my husband will testify to that! And people have an idea of what it looks like, and when I have my problems, they think, "Oh, she's drunk." Or, "Why is she holding on to that lamp-post?" and things.

Eventually, though, Jean said:

> I learned after a while to laugh at it because you realize how ridiculous it is. And I thought, you've got two choices, you either sit down and cry and feel sorry for yourself or you laugh. I did think of one good thing: there's one time when there was

a particular place you get off the bus and there's a lamppost, and I just hold it. And this old lady was giving me [a look] so I said to her, "It's all right, dear, I've just got a lamppost fetish." That wiped the smile off her face [laughing]! I don't always think of something like that. It's bad enough looking drunk if I was able to drink, but I can't cope with drink anyway [laughing]!

Jean's severely constrained ability to travel has meant that she doesn't go out as often as she might otherwise like, and she needs to carefully consider how she is going to get someplace. Sometimes, the location of something means that she simply can't go. When she first found out about meetings for people with stroke, for instance, she wasn't able to get there.

She felt isolated in her experience until she came across information about Different Strokes, a non-profit organization (called a charity in the UK) run by young people who've had a stroke, which holds regular meetings and offers support to young stroke survivors. The organization had only started holding meetings at the end of 1996, the same year Jean had her stroke. She learned about it after getting in touch with the more established Stroke Association. When a local group was organized, which included both exercise and social support group aspects, Jean became quite involved. She is enthusiastic about the importance of being able to get together with others who've shared a similar experience:

They're brilliant because to get to a whole lot of people and compare notes and — I mean, the exercise is, obviously very useful — but getting together with like people in the same boat and just finding out you're not the only one. I didn't know anybody who'd had one. I mean, whatever has happened to you, you discover when you say it to somebody, "Gosh, you wouldn't believe I thought this or I did this," and they say, "Oh yes, so did *I*." And you suddenly think you're not quite so crazy. And everybody swaps horror stories and funny stories. And we don't take ourselves too seriously; we have a lot of fun. It's every Saturday morning.

For a time, Jean volunteered as the local group's co-ordinator:

> When I first started, it was a lady called Joan who was the co-ordinator. And meeting *her* for the first time was one of the best things because here was a lady who was walking completely *normally*, speaking absolutely normally. And when she said hers was such a big stroke that she couldn't speak, she was in rehab for god knows how many months and couldn't speak *at all*, I thought, "Blimey, if she can do it ..." Everybody felt the same. And she was in charge for two years; then she moved, so I took over it for two years.

With the others at Different Strokes, Jean feels she is able to find a level of acceptance and understanding that is otherwise missing in her life. There are members of her family, for instance, who are sympathetic to her difficulties, but they can't really *understand* what it's like for Jean to cope with the residual effects of her stroke. As she said, "My brother and his wife, neither of them, bless them, have ever been ill. They can't quite understand what it's like. I don't think it's badness, I think it's incomprehension."

As Jean focused on recovery, she tried to put the idea of returning to the job she so disliked in the back of her mind. Jean was able to put off a decision about returning to work for a year. For the first six months after her stroke, she was receiving her full salary and for the next six months, she was on half salary. She was "terrified of having to go back to work and starting the whole sort of stress again." Indeed, she said that, "emotionally, I'd been such a mess before because of this job and everything. But in fact, by having a break from that, surprisingly, it was like a bit of a retreat."

When it came time for her to think about returning, she met with the occupational health specialist to discuss what she could do. Her impairments had been documented in reports that various therapists had written and sent to her employer. Especially given her memory problem and her shaky hands, everyone agreed that she couldn't return to her old job. (Jean also ended up letting go of her dream to become a massage therapist.) Someone suggested that she could work in the office, but Jean didn't think she was able to do that. Rather, Jean said, "I suggested scrubbing the floors as the only option." The specialist pointed out that she didn't have the balance to do that. Finally, it was decided that there were no jobs available that Jean could do and she should take early retirement. For Jean, this was welcome news:

> I didn't tell them that I had been in the process of trying to do something else and leave, they didn't know that. So when they said, "I'm afraid we're going to have to let you go," I resisted the temptation of leaping up, saying *yea*! I actually looked solemn as one should. And, I'll be honest, I had a great feeling of relief 'cause I'm sure stress was one of the reasons I had the stroke.

Not having to go back to work was probably the best thing that happened to Jean as a result of her stroke. She has never gone through a long period of depression on account of the stroke, although "there are moments I get very low." At such times, she has learned to cheer herself up by saying to herself, "If I hadn't had the stroke, where would I be now? Struggling down on the rush hour, working at that blasted place still [laughing]!" The stroke, then, represents a kind of freedom to Jean. She is quite happy with her post-stroke life: "I mean, sometimes I wish I could do a bit more, but you know, for all the struggling, I was just struggling and I'm not anymore. I just sort of thank god I can do the garden."

*

For Jean, life may have become more circumscribed than she would have wanted, but she is able to see the silver lining in the cloud. And she is always ready to laugh at herself when things aren't going as well as they could. With the support of her husband, her friends and her compatriot stroke survivors, Jean is thriving as she navigates post-stroke life. Accessing rehabilitation earlier would probably have been of great benefit to her, and she will likely always wonder how much more she would be able to do had it happened sooner, but she is so grateful for her music therapy that this positive rehabilitation experience outshines the negative.

Jean recently told me that she is "still going forward in my usual crooked way — I still don't 'do straight lines.'" As well, her husband has recently become disabled and has difficulty walking. Jean feels that she is better able to help him because of her own experiences of disability. She jokes: "Think of us as a pantomime horse — he does the head and I do the legs!"

Epilogue

By the time I embarked upon my "survivors project," I had already learned that my own experience of hemorrhagic stroke in childhood was not as rare as most people think. I knew that there were others out there somewhere who had been through similar experiences, and I wanted to know what they had to say about how their lives had been affected. I wanted to collect their stories so that I could contribute to the shattering of the destructive myth that stroke only happens to people over a certain age. Not only has it worked to prevent medical personnel from recognizing that a child or young adult has had a stroke, it has also worked to marginalize the experiences of those of us who have had a stroke in our youth. To talk about our experiences in mainstream society is to risk being misunderstood or, worse, regarded as alien. Thus, it is my hope that this book will help to open up space for women to talk about their experiences of surviving hemorrhagic stroke and that our voices will become part of the mainstream so we might feel a little less alien when we risk talking about these experiences that have so deeply shaped our lives.

In gathering these stories, not only did I meet and trade stories with eleven remarkable women, I also learned an enormous amount about how our experiences can be both similar and different. These stories about lives in process show us that not only are the impairments from hemorrhagic stroke devastating but so too are the psychological and emotional effects. In this regard, age is an especially important factor. In considering these women's stories, as well as my own, I think it is clear that, as much as the older women were affected, those of us who were children or young adults were affected in a different way. Deirdre and I, who both had a stroke before puberty, had not yet begun to make real plans about what we would do as adults, and there were no expectations after recovery that we should do anything other than continue to be children, with all of the dependency implied by that stage of life. Consequently, we were able to grow into adulthood having had the chance to incorporate, to a certain degree, knowledge about our impairments into a sense of ourselves.

Lauren and Liz, though still very young at seventeen years old, were on the cusp of adulthood. Both were eagerly planning what they would do when they left home. Both were excitedly anticipating the immanent arrival of adult independence. Consequently, both experienced the stroke as an exceptionally cruel blow. Similarly, Esther's entry into the world of adult independence was too recent for her to feel that she had had a chance to establish herself to her own satisfaction when she had her stroke. It is telling that all three women found that it took a very long time before they could feel able to move on with their lives in positive ways.

The other women profiled here had already had the chance to fully experience themselves as adults in control of their own lives when they had their strokes. This is in no way to suggest that the psychological impact was not as great as it was for those of us who were younger. By and large, though, these women did seem to adjust to their changed circumstances much more quickly than those who were younger. No doubt they were assisted by the fact that they had achieved a certain level of maturity borne of past experience.

Collectively, I think these stories show that the almost exclusive rehabilitative priority of functional ability is misplaced. Attention needs to be given to the psychological and emotional well-being of survivors and to preparing survivors to cope in the world beyond the hospital — in as timely a manner as physical rehabilitation allows. This means doing more than making sure that someone can walk unassisted. Minimally, survivors need to be made aware of potential impairments that may not become apparent until after they leave the hospital. This is particularly important for women, because we are typically socialized to take responsibility for things beyond our control and to blame ourselves when things do not go well. In this regard, there is a kind of similarity between a woman in an abusive relationship who thinks that she deserves no better and a woman who, for example, experiences profound fatigue on account of stroke but who nevertheless pushes herself to try harder to do more. If survivors are told how common it is to experience profound fatigue, they might be less likely to blame themselves for feeling tired. They might be more likely to be kind to themselves. It is all too common for women to push ourselves, to find ourselves imperfect and blame ourselves for our imperfections, perhaps because we see ourselves through the eyes of others. We need to stop judging ourselves by the standards of outsiders. This is easier said than done, though, and most of us are going to have a very hard time coming to this realization on our own. This is why it is vital to pay attention to the psychological and emotional well-being of survivors and to connect survivors with the professional expertise that is out there to help them.

These stories also show the extent to which there continues to be a bias towards recognizing visible impairment as disabling while discounting the significance of invisible impairment such as, for example, Jean Barton's poor balance or cognitive impairment, which is experienced by almost all of the women in this book. As discussed within the context of Ida King's story, few women ever receive any kind of cognitive rehabilitation. There is a tremendous silence surrounding the subject of cognitive impairment that needs to be broken. The silence means that when survivors experience difficulties, they are likely to blame themselves (as I did for decades) rather than seek help and support. More attention needs to be given to the possibility of cognitive impairment following hemorrhagic stroke. Medical personnel and rehabilitation professionals, in particular, need to better prepare their patients for life outside of a protected hospital environment.

Finally, the question might be asked: How representative are these women of the larger population of women who have a hemorrhagic stroke before the age of fifty? My answer is that they are certainly not representative of those who have been left with impairments so severe that they need ongoing assistance with personal care activities or of those who aren't able to accept that life with impairments can be a good life — those who suffer from treatment-resistant depression or who commit suicide. Nor are they representative of those who survive a hemorrhagic stroke with no impairments at all, or those who, because they have no residual impairment, do not consider their experiences to have lasting psychological ramifications. Such women exist, and with all the advances being made in the treatment of ruptured aneurysms and AVMs — new diagnostic tools, surgical advances and increasing awareness on the part of emergency personnel that strokes can and do happen to young people — it is becoming increasingly likely that the numbers of survivors with no residual impairment will grow. And last, but not least, they are not representative of those who live in abject poverty. Rehabilitation therapies can be expensive, and most of the assistance available requires a certain amount of financial input from the survivor. Similarly, even finding support can take a certain level of discretionary income — whether it be finding money to use public transit to get to a group or having Internet access to make use of resources on the Web.

There is precious little known about the long-term consequences of hemorrhagic stroke. What is clear from these stories is that everyone's journey is her own, and each one of us has recovered in remarkable ways. If the only thing someone knew about us was that we had survived a hemorrhagic stroke, then that someone would know hardly anything about us. But these stories also seem to paint a broader picture about what can be helpful in recovery. Themes that recur throughout include strong goals (such as those relating to career or education), excellent support (from friends, family, community and professionals), good rehabilitation, creative problem-solving and strong identity and beliefs (whether it's one's attitude, self-esteem or religious faith). Not to mention the chance to talk about one's experience.

A stroke is, in a curious way, an amazing thing. It can so utterly debilitate us physically, mentally and spiritually, but it can also be seen as a kind of metaphor for people's amazing ability to recover, heal, adapt and accept. Stroke is not necessarily an unmitigated tragedy. The women who've shared their stories here are all testament to that.

Glossary

AFO (Ankle-Foot Orthoses): An orthoses is a brace. An AFO is worn to help stabilize walking.

Aneurysm: A brain aneurysm is a bulge of the wall of a blood vessel in the brain. It is a weakening in the wall with a propensity to rupture. Also known as a cerebral aneurysm, the bulge may pose little risk to health as long as it is small and doesn't rupture. An aneurysm may go undetected indefinitely and produce no signs or symptoms. However, some brain aneurysms are large enough to put pressure on surrounding brain tissue. Others may rupture at a weak spot in the artery wall and flood an area of the brain with blood (hemorrhage). A ruptured aneurysm can quickly become life-threatening and requires prompt medical attention. People of all ages can have a brain aneurysm, but most are discovered in people ages thirty-five to sixty. Women are slightly more likely than men to develop an aneurysm.

Aneurysm Treatments:

1. *Clipping:* This is the most common treatment for an aneurysm. A tiny clamp is placed at the base of the aneurysm, isolating it from the circulation of the artery to which it's attached. This can keep the aneurysm from bursting, or it can prevent re-bleeding of an aneurysm that has recently hemorrhaged.

2. *Endovascular Embolization (also known as coiling):* In an embolization procedure, a catheter is maneuvered into the aneurysm. A tiny platinum coil is pushed through the catheter and positioned inside the aneurysm. The coil fills the aneurysm, causing clotting and sealing the aneurysm off from connecting arteries. This is a relatively new procedure (since the 1990s).

Angiogram (also known as arteriogram): An imaging test that uses X-rays to view blood vessels. This is the definitive method to detect aneurysms. Using a groin artery, a catheter is placed in the blood vessels leading to the brain and a contrast agent or dye is injected to give detailed pictures of the blood vessels.

AVM (Arteriovenous Malformation): An AVM is a tangle of abnormal and poorly formed blood vessels (arteries and veins). They have a higher rate of bleeding than normal vessels. AVMs can occur anywhere in the body. Brain

AVMs are of special concern because of the damage they cause when they bleed. They can occur in any part of the brain. It is a congenital disorder (present at birth). The cause of an AVM isn't clear.

AVM Treatments:

1. *Embolization:* Under general anaesthesia, a small catheter (plastic tube) is advanced from the groin into the brain vessels and then into the AVM. A non-reactive liquid glue is injected into the vessels which form the AVM to block off the AVM. There is a small risk to this procedure and the chances of completely curing the AVM using this technique depend on the size of the AVM. It is frequently combined with other treatments such as radiation or surgery.

2. *Radiosurgery:* This treatment is also known as Radiation Treatment or Stereotactic Radiotherapy. A narrow x-ray beam is focused on the AVM such that a high dose is concentrated on the AVM with a much lower dose delivered to the rest of the brain. This radiation causes the AVM to shrivel up and close off over a period of 2-3 years in up to 80% of patients. The risk of complications is low. Until the AVM is completely closed off, the risk of bleeding still persists.

Aphasia: An impairment of the ability to use or comprehend words, usually acquired as a result of a stroke or other brain injury. There are three main types of aphasia:

1. *Broca's aphasia*: An inability to express language and articulate sentences correctly. Speech tends to be non-fluent, minimal or disjointed and grammar is impaired, but comprehension is not greatly affected. Reading and writing can also be affected.

2. *Wernicke's aphasia*: Difficulty in understanding language, despite retaining normal intelligence in other ways. People with Wernicke's aphasia talk fluently and grammatically, but the content is garbled or nonsensical. These people may speak in long sentences that have no meaning, add unnecessary words, or even create new words. Reading and writing can also be impaired.

3. *Global aphasia*: Damage to extensive portions of the brain. Results in severe communication difficulties and may limit a person's ability to speak or comprehend language.

Botox (Botulinum toxin): Botox is a biological product injected into specific muscles where it acts to reduce the involuntary contractions that cause the symptoms of dystonia. The injections weaken muscle activity sufficiently to reduce a spasm but not enough to cause paralysis. Because the effect wears off, injections (which are painful) need to be repeated approximately every three months.

Cavernous malformation: A vascular abnormality of the central nervous system. It consists of a cluster of abnormal, dilated vessels.

Cognitive impairment: Cognitive impairment can affect the ability to understand and/or use language (see aphasia), reasoning, judgement or intuition. It can affect the ability to read, write or otherwise focus on something, and it can affect memory. Survivors of hemorrhagic stroke commonly find that their short-term memory has been negatively affected.

Coma: A state of prolonged unconsciousness in which the brain functions at its lowest level of alertness. A person in a coma cannot be awakened and does not respond purposefully to physical or verbal stimulation. Occasionally a doctor may induce a coma with drugs to protect the brain and give it a chance to heal after brain surgery. Doctors may also induce a coma when someone is experiencing prolonged seizures or to control brain swelling caused by a brain injury from head trauma, a stroke or an infection.

CT scan (Computerized Tomography): A CT scan uses X-rays to image different parts of the body. CT scanning is an excellent method of detecting bleeding into the brain or the fluid spaces around the brain. The study of the brain may be done either with or without dye. On the CT scan, it may be possible to see evidence of hemorrhage associated with a brain aneurysm.

Dystonia: Dystonia is a neurological movement disorder characterized by involuntary, sustained muscle contractions, which force certain parts of the body into abnormal, sometimes painful, movements or postures. It is the third most common neurological disorder after Parkinson's disease and tremor, affecting at least 200,000 persons in North America.

Dystonia Treatments:

1. Aside from botox injections, physical therapy is commonly used to treat dystonia. A common phenomenon associated with dystonia is called a sensory trick, or *geste antagoniste*. Touching an affected or adjacent body part can sometimes significantly reduce contractions. For example, placing a hand on the chin, side of the face or back of the head may reduce neck muscle contractions. People with dystonia typically discover this and use this trick to reduce their own dystonic contractions. Some physical therapists have developed head or neck braces, hand splints or other devices that mimic the sensory trick.

2. A physical therapist may also recommend stretches and exercises that enhance flexibility and range of motion, strengthen underutilized muscles and promote optimal posture. The therapist may identify movements or activities that exacerbate dystonia symptoms and help to develop methods to avoid those movements.

EEG (Electroencephalogram): In this painless test, electrodes are placed on the scalp to measure electrical activity produced by the brain. An EEG can diagnose epilepsy and determine what type of seizures are occurring. It can also identify the location of a suspected brain tumor, inflammation, infection, bleeding, head injury or disease in the brain.

Embolization. See Aneurysm Treatments and AVM Treatments.

Epilepsy/Epileptic seizures: Epilepsy is a chronic disorder of the brain that causes a tendency to have recurrent seizures. Two or more seizures must occur before a person can receive the diagnosis of epilepsy, also known as a seizure disorder. Seizures occur when there's a sudden change in the normal way brain cells communicate through electrical signals. During a seizure, some brain cells send abnormal signals, which stop other cells from working properly. This abnormality may cause temporary changes in sensation, behaviour, movement or consciousness.

Having a seizure can result in the sudden occurrence of any activity that is co-ordinated by the brain. This can include temporary confusion, complete loss of consciousness, a staring spell or uncontrollable, jerking movements of the arms and legs. Signs and symptoms may vary depending on the type of seizure. Most people with epilepsy experience the same type of seizure, with similar symptoms, each time they have a seizure, but some may experience a wide range of types and symptoms.

Types of Epileptic Seizures:

1. *Simple partial seizures:* These seizures begin from a small area in the brain and do not result in loss of consciousness. They may cause uncontrolled shaking of an arm, leg or any other part of the body; alter emotions; change the way things look, smell, feel, taste or sound; or cause speech disturbance.

2. *Complex partial seizures:* These seizures also begin from a small area of the brain. They alter consciousness and usually cause memory loss (amnesia). They can cause staring and non-purposeful movements, such as repeated hand rubbing, lip smacking, posturing of the arm, vocalization or swallowing. After the seizure ends, the person may be confused or sleep for a few minutes and may be unaware of having had the seizure.

3. *Secondary generalized seizures (partial seizures with secondary generalization):* These seizures occur when simple or complex seizures spread to involve the entire brain. They may begin as a complex partial seizure with staring and non-purposeful movements. The seizure then becomes more intense, leading to generalized convulsions characterized by stiffening and shaking of the extremities and the body with loss of consciousness.

4. *Petit mal seizures (absence):* These seizures are characterized by staring, subtle body movement and brief lapses of awareness. They are usually brief and typically no confusion or sleepiness occurs when the seizure is over.

5. *Myoclonic seizures:* These seizures usually appear as sudden jerks of the arms and legs. Myoclonic seizures may last only a short time — from less than a second for single jerks to a few seconds for repeated jerks.

6. *Atonic seizures:* Also known as drop attacks, these seizures cause one to suddenly collapse or fall down. After a few seconds, the person regains consciousness and is able to stand and walk.

7. *Grand mal seizures (generalized tonic-clonic):* The most intense of all types of seizures, these are characterized by a loss of consciousness, body stiffening and shaking, and sometimes tongue biting or loss of bladder control. After the shaking subsides, a period of confusion or sleepiness usually occurs, lasting for a few minutes to a few hours.

Grand mal seizures: See Types of Epileptic Seizures.

Hemiplegia (also known as hemiparesis): A condition involving paralysis or partial paralysis of one side of the body. Signs of hemiplegia include muscle weakness or stiffness (spasticity); paralysis on one side; lack of control on the affected side of the body; little use of one hand; limping, toe drop, gait problems; poor balance; speech or language difficulties; and visual field defects.

Hemorrhagic stroke: Hemorrhage is the medical word for bleeding. Hemorrhagic stroke occurs when a blood vessel in the brain leaks or ruptures. Hemorrhages can result from a number of conditions that affect blood vessels, including uncontrolled high blood pressure (hypertension) and weak spots in blood vessel walls (aneurysms). A less common cause of hemorrhage is the rupture of an arteriovenous malformation (AVM) — a malformed tangle of thin-walled blood vessels, present at birth. The two types of hemorrhagic stroke are intracerebral hemorrhage and subarachnoid hemorrhage.

Hydrocephalus: Hydrocephalus comes from the Greek *hydro*, which means "water", and *cephalus*. which means "head". Hydrocephalus is an abnormal accumulation of cerebrospinal fluid (CSF) within cavities called ventricles inside the brain. As the CSF builds up, it causes the ventricles to enlarge and the pressure inside the head to increase (fluid buildup in the brain; brain swelling).
The most common method of treating hydrocephalus is the surgical placement of a shunt. A shunt is a flexible tube placed into the ventricular system that diverts the flow of CSF into another region of the body where it can be absorbed, such as the peritoneal (abdominal) cavity or the right atrium of the heart. The shunt tube is about 1/8 inch in diameter and is made of a soft and pliable plastic that is well tolerated by our body tissues. Shunt systems come in a variety of models but have similar functional components. Catheters (tubing) and a flow-control mechanism (one-way valve) are components common to all shunts. The valve in the shunt maintains the CSF at normal pressure within the ventricles.

Intracerebral hemorrhage: In this type of stroke, a blood vessel in the brain bursts and spills into the surrounding brain tissue, damaging cells. Brain cells beyond the leak are deprived of blood and are also damaged. High blood pressure is the most common cause of this type of hemorrhagic stroke. High blood pressure can cause small arteries inside the brain to become brittle and susceptible to cracking and rupture.

Ischemic stroke: About 80% of strokes are ischemic. They occur when blood clots or other particles block arteries to the brain and cause severely reduced blood flow (ischemia). This deprives the brain cells of oxygen and nutrients, and cells may begin to die within minutes.

Lumbar puncture: A lumbar puncture, also called a spinal tap, removes a small amount of cerebrospinal fluid (CSF) — the fluid that protects the brain and spinal cord from injury — for laboratory analysis. The test also measures the pressure in CSF fluid. Results of a lumbar puncture can help diagnose bleeding around the brain (subarachnoid hemorrhage).

MRI (Magnetic Resonance Imaging): A special imaging technique used to image internal structures of the body, particularly the soft tissues. An MRI image is often superior to a normal X-ray image. Images are very clear and are particularly good for soft tissue, brain and spinal cord, joints and abdomen.

Neuropsychologists: The primary activity of neuropsychologists is to assess brain functioning through structured and systematic behavioural observation. Neuropsychological tests are designed to examine a variety of cognitive abilities, including speed of information processing, attention, memory, language and executive functions, which are necessary for goal-directed behaviour. By testing a range of cognitive abilities and examining patterns of performance in different cognitive areas, neuropsychologists can make inferences about underlying brain function.

Petit mal seizures. See Types of Epileptic Seizures.

Radiosurgery. See AVM Treatments.

Subarachnoid hemorrhage: In this type of stroke, bleeding starts in a large artery on or near the membrane surrounding the brain and spills into the space between the surface of the brain and the skull. It specifically occurs within the cerebrospinal fluid-filled spaces surrounding the brain (also known as the subarachnoid space). A subarachnoid hemorrhage is often signalled by a sudden, severe "thunderclap" headache. This type of stroke is commonly caused by the rupture of an aneurysm. After a subarachnoid hemorrhage, vessels may go into vasospasm, a condition in which arteries near the hemorrhage constrict erratically, causing brain cell damage by further restricting or blocking blood flow to portions of the brain.

Shunt. See Hydrocephalus.

Tracheotomy: A surgical procedure in which an incision is made in the front of the neck and a breathing tube is inserted through a hole (stoma) into the windpipe (trachea). Breathing then takes place through the tube, bypassing the immobilized vocal cords.

Vasospasm: A narrowing of the arteries that can lead to lack of blood flow to part of the brain (an ischemic stroke).

Vertigo: Vertigo is the sudden sensation of being unsteady, or that surroundings are moving. One may feel as though they are spinning around or that the head is spinning inside. The condition is characterized by brief episodes of intense dizziness associated with a change in the position of the head. It may occur when moving the head in a certain direction, lying down from an upright position, turning over in bed or sitting up in the morning. Moving the head to look up can also bring about an episode of vertigo. Vertigo usually results from a problem with the nerves and the structures of the balance mechanism in the inner ear that sense movement and changes in the position of the head.

* The following Internet sources were used in the compilation of this glossary:
Aphasia Hope Foundation (www.aphasiahope.org/faq.jsp);
Children's Hemiplegia & Stroke Association (www.chasa.org);
Dystonia Medical Research Foundation (www.dystonia-foundation.org);
Healthline (www.healthline.com); Hydrocephalus Association
(www.hydroassoc.org); Mayo Clinic (www.mayoclinic.com); Toronto Brain
Vascular Malformation Study Group (brainavm.oci.utoronto.ca);
and WebMD (www.webmd.com).

Selected Internet Resources

American Stroke Association

www.strokeassociation.org/presenter.jhtml?identifier=1200037

Offers a broad range of information on pediatric stroke and an online support group/discussion board. American residents can subscribe to the highly rated *Stroke Connection* magazine, which contains survivor stories, tips on living with stroke and information about research and rehabilitation. Excerpts from *Stroke Connection* are published on the website. Highly recommended.

AVM Support UK

www.avmsupport.org.uk/

This site offers information about AVMs along with online support.

Aneurysm & AVM Support (U.S.)

www.westga.edu/~wmaples/aneurysm.html

Established in 1995 by Bill Maples who is associated with the University of West Georgia, this site contains an amazing collection of narratives written by people who have been diagnosed with an aneurysm or AVM (some hemorrhaged, some did not). New narratives are continually being posted. My own "Childhood Aneurysm" was posted on the Aneurysms page on September 16, 1996, which was before the page for AVMs was created. As well, there are links to a wealth of medical information. Highly recommended.

Aphasia Hope Foundation (U.S.)

www.aphasiahope.org/faq.jsp

Contains an abundance of information and research about aphasia and on living with aphasia. Highly recommended.

Children's Hemiplegia & Stroke Association (U.S.)

www.chasa.org

Offers a great selection of information about childhood hemiplegia and an e-mail support group for families.

Different Strokes (UK)

www.differentstrokes.co.uk/

This is the website for the UK-based organization Different Strokes, which is run by young stroke survivors for young stroke survivors. There is a broad selection of information about stroke, a growing number of survivor stories, an active message board (mostly UK participants, but some are international) and the quarterly newsletter, which can be downloaded. The newsletter is also available by regular mail. Highly recommended.

Generation S: Young Stroke Survivors (U.S.)

www.orgsites.com/pa/generation-s

An interesting website run by a survivor and his partner in Pittsburgh, Pennsylvania, although it does not appear to have been updated for several years.

Heart and Stroke Foundation (Canada)

ww2.heartandstroke.ca/Page.asp?PageID=1017&CategoryID=2&Src=stroke

A wealth of information about stroke and living with the consequences of stroke. Highly recommended.

National Stroke Association (U.S.)

www.stroke.org

This site offers a broad range of information about stroke. American residents can subscribe to the highly rated *Stroke Smart* magazine, which contains survivor stories, tips on living with stroke and information about research and rehabilitation.

Pediatric Stroke Network (U.S.)

www.pediatricstrokenetwork.com

Offers a wealth of information about childhood stroke. Highly recommended.

SAFE: Stroke Awareness for Everyone (U.S.)

www.strokesafe.org

Offers online support and information for stroke survivors and caregivers. Provides a very good list of resources.

StrokeNet, A Stroke Support Community (U.S.)

www.strokenetwork.org/

An online stroke support and information group for stroke survivors and caregivers, this site offers a very active and welcoming message board involving many participants from a variety of countries around the world. Participants are mostly non-elderly. The site also offers a monthly e-mail newsletter. Highly recommended.

Stroke Survivors Association of Ottawa (Canada)

www.strokesurvivors.ca

Offers a broad selection of information about stroke and living with the consequences of stroke, and is aimed at survivors of all ages.

Subarachnoid Hemorrhage (UK)

www.srht.nhs.uk/patient--visitor-information/services-support/sub-arachnoid-haemorrhage/

This page is embedded within the website for the Salford Royal NHS Foundation Trust. It was created by medical and nursing teams from the Wessex and Greater Manchester Neuroscience Centres and contains a wealth of information about subarachnoid hemorrhage. It is well worth typing in the rather complex URL to take a look at all it offers. Highly recommended.

The Goddess Fund (U.S.)

www.thegoddessfund.org

A very interesting website intended to raise awareness about stroke in women. There is information about women and stroke, and there are survivor stories on the site.

The National Aphasia Association (U.S.)

www.aphasia.org

The NAA's mission is to educate the public to know that the word aphasia describes an impairment of the ability to communicate, not an impairment of intellect. The website offers much information about recovering from or compensating for aphasia. Especially noteworthy is the Young People's Network page at www.aphasia.org/ aphasia_community/young_peoples_network.html.

The Toronto Brain Vascular Malformation Study Group (Canada)

http://brainavm.uhnres.utoronto.ca/brainavm/servlet/main?flash=true

This website is sponsored by the Toronto Western Hospital (University of Toronto). It contains of a great deal of information about brain aneurysms, AVMs and other brain malformations, and treatment options. There is also a support page.